# THE FLAT HEAD SYNDROME FIX

*A Parent's Guide to Simple and Surprising Strategies for Preventing Plagiocephaly and Rounding Out Baby's Flat Spots Without a Helmet*

RACHEL COLEY, MS, OT/L

Published by CanDo Kiddo, LLC
November, 2015

For permission requests, please email the publisher at rachel@candokiddo.com

# CONTENTS

# YOU'RE WORRIED ABOUT FLAT HEAD SYNDROME

Let's face it, since you found out you were pregnant, you've worried about a LOT of things. Keeping your little one's head round and avoiding a baby helmet is just one of the many.

Research shows that *nearly 50% of babies will experience head flattening*[22] and that there are some negative long-term consequences of Flat Head Syndrome. In this case, it seems your worrying isn't totally misplaced (as it is when you lay in bed awake at night fretting about whether your baby's ingrown toenail might lead to a massive infection and eventual amputation).

**Here's the good news** – by following the simple strategies in this book, you'll give your baby the best chance possible of being in the 50% of babies with a round head. The knowledge and tools you're about to receive will equip you to reduce your baby's risk of ending up wearing a helmet. And the steps you'll take to prevent and manage Flat Head Syndrome will give your baby the healthiest start possible.

The even better news is that by spreading the word and sharing the resource you hold in your hands, you can become a vital piece of *The Flat Head Syndrome Fix* and help reduce that 50% statistic. Help your baby and help other babies – does it get any more rewarding than that?

# WE CAN FIX THAT! HERE'S HOW I KNOW...

---

**The Flat Head Syndrome Fix has the potential to prevent or reduce the severity of head flattening in babies.**

How do I know? Because I've seen it work.

I've seen flat spots disappear. Heads round out. Helmets avoided.

I've seen prevention keep heads round. Promote healthy development. Avoid long-term complications.

And I've seen parents go from worried to confident. From survival mode to strategic. From feeling helpless to feeling empowered.

Since 2006, I've worked with thousands of families as a pediatric Occupational Therapist. Together, we've implemented simple, realistic strategies and tools to improve the health and development of their children. I've also scribbled down notes, sketched treatment ideas and drunk gallons of coffee in hundreds of hours of courses about infant development, head shape and neck issues of infancy.

*I see no reason why the tools that parents need to prevent and reduce the severity of Flat Head Syndrome should be confined to courses for therapists or to clinics.* The parents who desperately want and need this information deserve to have it. And I'm excited to share it with you.

Let's take this flat head worry off your plate so that you can focus more attention on enjoying your adorable baby.

Rachel Coley, MS, OT/L
Occupational Therapist
Founder of CanDoKiddo.com

# WHAT IS THE FLAT HEAD SYNDROME FIX?

You're probably thinking, "Alright, show me the Fix! Give me the tools and strategies! Let's do this thing!" I appreciate your eagerness and I can totally understand your impulse to skip ahead to the juicy parts.

But I need you to hang with me for a few chapters so that we can fully understand what's really behind the Flat Head Syndrome epidemic. These first few chapters make up Part One of the four-part *Flat Head Syndrome Fix*.

**Part One: "Debunking Flat Head Syndrome Myths"**
**Understanding the problem**

There are some things we've been led to believe about Flat Head Syndrome that aren't fully true and aren't helpful. Your baby can do hours of Tummy Time a day, but if you don't fully understand what *really* causes Flat Head Syndrome, your sweet babe might still be on the road to wearing a helmet.

The first step to fixing any problem is really understanding the problem. I know too many parents who've only come to a clearer understanding of head flattening once their baby has it. Even then, many have their babies' head shapes treated but don't walk away from the experience with clear, comprehensive information about how to prevent, detect and manage head flattening.

By the time you're finished with Part One of this book, you'll arrive at those tips, tools and strategies you're craving with a more thorough understanding of Flat Head Syndrome. I can also almost guarantee that you will have learned something new. My hope is that you'll find what you learn so surprising that you won't be able to keep it to yourself. You can be a part of a widespread *Flat Head Syndrome Fix* by sharing your newfound greater understanding of Flat Head Syndrome within your circle of influence.

**Part Two: "My Baby's Head Is Round – Isn't It?"**
**Early detection of Flat Head Syndrome**

An essential part of *The Flat Head Syndrome Fix* – oh, who am I kidding? All four parts are completely essential. I tried hard not to put anything in this book that isn't essential because we both have diapers to change and laundry to do. But early detection is really, really (really) important.

The earlier head flattening is noticed, the earlier you can make the simple changes to stop and hopefully reverse it. Earlier treatments are more effective and decrease the chances that a helmet will be recommended for your baby a few months down the road. Noticing that your baby's head is getting just a little flat can result in less chance of your little one experiencing the long-term health and developmental effects associated with Flat Head Syndrome that we'll discuss in Part One.

**Part Three: "Keep It Round"**
**Preventing Flat Head Syndrome**

In Part Three of this book, we'll take a deep dive into preventing Flat Head Syndrome. Based on my experience as a pediatric OT and mom, I've put together a simple way of thinking about your baby's positioning that any new parent can use to help prevent Flat Head Syndrome. As an added bonus, these prevention efforts, which I call **Proactive Positioning**, will promote your baby's healthy overall development. Parenting wins can be few and far between in the newborn days. A plan that prevents Flat Head Syndrome *and* promotes motor skills, milestones and learning? That's the new parent equivalent of a buy one, get three free deal on diapers!

If your baby already shows signs of head flattening, you might be tempted to skip Part Three of this book. Please don't. It lays an important framework for *The Flat Head Syndrome Fix* that will make Part Four even more effective. We'll get to your Fix in no time, I promise.

**Part Four: "Round It Back Out"**
**Stop the flattening and reshape your baby's head**

Guess who has the biggest potential to change the shape of your baby's head? Not your pediatrician, not a helmet provider, not a chiropractor, but YOU! Now, that can feel empowering and you probably charge yourself a much lower fee than those other providers. But it can also feel overwhelming. Don't panic. I'll walk you through the simple changes you can make to your baby's daily routines to stop head flattening in its tracks and give your baby the best chance of head re-shaping without using a helmet.

Flat Head Syndrome isn't *always* avoidable. Despite your diligent efforts to implement the strategies, tools and tips of *The Flat Head Syndrome Fix*, you may still face the daunting decision of whether or not to get a helmet for your baby. Talk about stressful! I'll help walk you through some important considerations, questions to ask and tools to guide your decision-making. With all the knowledge and data you'll have about your baby's head shape after reading this book, you'll feel more confident in whatever decision you make.

Are you ready to discover the power that you have to influence your baby's head shape? Are you eager to learn the strategies you can implement starting today to prevent Flat Head Syndrome, stop existing head flattening from getting worse or reshape your baby's head? If so, I'm ready to let you in on the best kept secrets in Flat Head Syndrome management. Let's get started!

# IMPORTANT DISCLAIMERS

Screech! Put on the brakes. There are just a few nitty gritty details that I need to put on the table before we proceed.

**This book will NOT address the identification or treatment of Craniosynostosis.** In this book, we'll be talking extensively about Flat Head Syndrome, but it's important to recognize that there is also a more serious, rare condition called Craniosynostosis that also results in atypical head shapes. Craniosynostosis involves the premature closure of the cranial sutures (skull joints), which is a serious condition requiring specialized care and, often, surgery. I know, one more scary condition to worry about! But take a deep breath on this one. Examining a baby's head for signs of Craniosynostosis is a routine part of a newborn exam in the hospital as well as early well-baby check-ups. Rest assured, if your child's care team suspects this condition you'll be referred promptly to a specialist.

**This book is intended for informational purposes only and is not intended to be a replacement for medical advice from a physician or other licensed health care provider.** Please consult your child's pediatrician if you suspect any medical or developmental issues with your child. The recommendations in this book are not intended to replace or override any individualized treatment plan from a health care provider based on his or her professional evaluation of an individual child. The recommendations in this book are based on current published research and the clinical education and experience of the author. They are no guarantee of results. Neither the author or CanDo Kiddo, LLC is liable for any injury incurred while implementing recommendations found within this book.

**The recommendations in this book are intended for the prevention and management of Flat Head Syndrome WHILE FOLLOWING the Back to Sleep / Safe to Sleep recommendations put forth by the National Institute of Child Health and Human Development and the American Academy of Pediatrics for the reduction of Sudden Infant Death Syndrome.** Some parents may choose alternative sleep positions, sleep environments or the use of sleep props for positioning their infants to prevent or treat head flattening. Some health care providers may make recommendations that are not in 100% compliance with Back to Sleep / Safe to Sleep guidelines. Individual family decisions about baby sleep should be made with full understanding of the risks and benefits after communication with a child's doctor.

Phew! Okay, now that we've gotten those out of the way...

PART I.

---

# DEBUNKING FLAT HEAD SYNDROME MYTHS

---

# CHAPTER 1.

## MYTH: HEAD SHAPE IS PURELY ABOUT APPEARANCE

---

It can be easy to assume that head shape is just a matter of appearance. Maybe you wonder if your baby's head shape will even matter once her hair grows. Many parents aren't alarmed at the first signs of flattening because they're reassured by friends, family and even their child's doctor that "it doesn't look that bad."

It's time to debunk the myth that Flat Head Syndrome is purely a cosmetic issue. I'm convinced that once a light is shown on the facts about the potential long-term effects of head flattening, you'll be ready to start *today* making the simple changes needed to help reduce your baby's risk of head flattening. And you won't be able to keep what you've learned to yourself. Why?

*I know that you and all of the parents you know want what's best for your babies.* You wouldn't be reading this book if you didn't. The fact that you frequently ask Google, read blogs, subscribe to parenting magazines and ask Google a few more times about issues related to your baby's health and development is a sure sign that you want more information. You want advice from infant experts and you want to know the steps to take to do what's best for your baby. You don't want myths, you want the truth. So here it is:

## 6 Reasons Why Your Baby's Head Shape Matters:

*Flattening of the head may be a red flag that your baby has muscle tightness.* Muscle tightness is very common in infants. Spotting and addressing tightness early on reduces the risk that it will cause long-term developmental problems such as motor delays.[8,12]

*Head flattening may be an early warning that your baby's movement is being restricted.* Head flattening is often the proverbial canary in the coal mine that can let parents know that their baby needs more variety in his daily positioning. Experiencing a wide variety of positions is critical for optimal motor, sensory and cognitive development and babies with head flattening show higher rates of developmental delays.[18,24,26]

*Head flattening can be an important signal of developmental problems.* Occasionally, head flattening can point to an underlying issue with muscle tone, vision, sensory processing and more. Early intervention for these challenges can reduce their severity and long-term complications.

*Head flattening and related facial asymmetry can result in lifelong jaw issues.*[16,31]

*Head flattening and related facial asymmetry can contribute to vision problems.*[30]

*Head flattening and related facial asymmetry can increase your child's risk of ear infections.*[28]

CHAPTER 2.

# MYTH: THE BACK TO SLEEP CAMPAIGN IS TO BLAME

---

If you've heard of Flat Head Syndrome, odds are that you've also heard that it's due to the Back to Sleep Campaign. It feels good to have a simple, clear cut cause for such an increasingly common problem, doesn't it? Oh boy, I hate to burst that bubble but I have to so that we can come to a shared understanding of what isn't such a simple problem and come closer to a fix. The good news is that by debunking this myth, we'll begin to more clearly see a path toward solutions.

The Back to Sleep campaign has played a key role in reducing the rates of Sudden Infant Death Syndrome by at least 40%.[2] I'm not willing to risk challenging or defying such an important infant safety mandate, are you? So if we continue to buy into the myth that the rise of Flat Head Syndrome is all due to the Back to Sleep Campaign, we can begin to feel pretty helpless, and finding a fix for head flattening seems hopeless.

It's true that sleeping on the back increases chances for Flat Head Syndrome to develop. But the whole truth is that there are many, many other contributing factors to head flattening.[29] By focusing on the one element that's nearly impossible to safely change, we miss the boat and overlook important opportunities for preventing and managing head shape problems.

There are strategies parents can use to try to influence their babies' head positions during sleep, which I'll describe in this book. But I'll also share all the ways that you can affect your babies' head shape during her wakeful times.[13] *Positioning strategies like those I'll describe in detail in this book have helped thousands of parents prevent, reverse and reduce the severity of Flat Head Syndrome – all while continuing to follow Back to Sleep recommendations.*

# CHAPTER 3.

## MYTH: MORE TUMMY TIME IS THE SOLUTION

---

As a pediatric Occupational Therapist, I'll join the chorus of people you've heard sing the praises of Tummy Time and its amazing developmental benefits for your baby. But I'm also going to let you in on a big secret (and give you permission and encouragement to share this secret). Increasing Tummy Time is one facet of *The Flat Head Syndrome Fix*, but it isn't the whole solution. Not by a long shot.

The combined myths that the Back to Sleep Campaign is the problem and that more Tummy Time is the solution neglect a really important fact about your baby's head that will be key to preventing and managing Flat Head Syndrome. Can you guess what it is?

It's the fact that your baby's head is round. Pretty important, right? Tummy Time is great (really, keep doing it!) and eliminates the pressure on the back of the head that baby gets when he's asleep, but your baby could do Tummy Time every single waking minute of his day and still get a flat head. That's because it doesn't address what *really* causes and fixes Flat Head Syndrome…

CHAPTER 4.

# MYTH: THE "WAIT AND SEE" APPROACH WORKS

You probably know some parents who noticed their baby's head getting flat and were told by their child's doctor, "let's wait and see what it looks like at their next appointment." Maybe you've even been told this. Very often, parents who receive this response leave the doctor's office feeling uneasy, with a gut feeling that there has to be *something* that they can do in the meantime.

That gut feeling? It's spot-on. With all due respect to primary care doctors and pediatricians, most don't receive comprehensive training in Flat Head Syndrome and many aren't up to date with current clinical guidelines for effective treatment.[5,19,27] *The "Wait and See" Approach is in complete opposition to the conclusion of nearly every single research study of effective treatments for head flattening.*[6,17] Time and time again, implementing repositioning strategies like those described in this book at a very early age has been shown to be the biggest factor in reducing the severity of head flattening and avoiding long-term complications (not to mention avoiding a helmet).

*Without specific guidance for changing a baby's daily routines using repositioning strategies, "Wait and See" effectively means 'let's wait and watch it stay the same or get worse."* As you learn the full story about what really affects your baby's head shape, you'll begin to see that without changing how your baby spends her day, the chances of significant spontaneous improvements in head shape are slim.

I'm here to take that gut feeling that parents have – that there must be *something* they can do – and give you the plan that can fix your baby's Flat Head problem.

# CHAPTER 5.

# A WORD ABOUT GUILT

---

Before we jump right into looking at what flattens heads, we need to talk about a pesky little feeling that might crop up as you read – GUILT. Becoming a parent strengthens our guilt muscles faster than Crossfit. I'm going to invite you to do what might seem like a silly exercise before we move on. But it's important. Please read the next lines out loud.

*I have always tried to do what's best for my child to the best of my knowledge. When I know more than I did before, it helps me be a better parent.*

Did you say it? I'm serious, I'll wait.

Why is this so important? Because as I discuss all the things you can do to prevent and manage Flat Head Syndrome, your guilty parent brain is probably hearing at least part of the information as "should haves," or "shouldn't haves." You might have a tendency to focus on looking back, but I assure you that the Fix lies in looking forward. Focus not on what you would do if you had a time machine, but on what you can start doing today to give your baby the healthiest start possible.

# CHAPTER 6.

# THE TRUTH ABOUT WHAT FLATTENS HEADS

If the Back to Sleep Campaign isn't solely to blame for head flattening, what else is? Let's take a look at why your baby's head is so moldable and examine some of the biggest factors that contribute to head flattening.

An infant's adorable little head is made up of a handful of large bones that haven't fully hardened yet, joined by flexible joints that act like expansion joints. The result is your baby's head having a consistency much more like an elementary schooler's wet paper-mâché project than a marble sculpture in a museum.

*In the vast majority of cases, Flat Head Syndrome results from a combination of factors within our control and those beyond our control.*[2,15,32] *There is usually no single cause that can be isolated (and no single person can be blamed).*

**Unpreventable Factors That Increase Risk of Head Flattening:**

- being first-born
- being a boy
- vacuum or forceps-assisted delivery
- prematurity (earlier than 37 weeks)

- multiple births (twins, triplets, etc.)
- congenital Torticollis (baby is born with)
- average to difficult baby temperament
- decreased movement in the womb
- breech positioning in the womb

**Preventable Factors That Increase Risk of Head Flattening:**

- increased time spent on the back (including sleep time *and* awake time)
- decreased activity and movement of a baby
- less than 1 hour daily spent upright
- Tummy Time less than 3 times per day
- head not repositioned at sleep times
- exclusive bottle feeding in one position
- untreated or unresolved Torticollis (neck tightness)

*Ultimately, the most important thing to understand is that the cause of head flattening is PRESSURE on the skull.* Whether baby is awake or asleep, not-yet-born or newly arrived in the world, pressure molds the head. Whether that pressure comes from mommy's pelvic bone in the womb, from a mattress or from daddy's arm when held, pressure causes head flattening.

If pressure is the cause of head flattening, then you're probably wondering what's the key to preventing or fixing it?

# CHAPTER 7.

# THE REAL KEY TO FIGHTING FLAT HEAD SYNDROME

The key to fixing head flattening in babies? Pressure. Yes, **the very same thing that causes flattening is the key ingredient in The Flat Head Syndrome Fix**. Take a moment to let that sink in – the solution to the problem lives right there in the cause of it. As it turns out, pressure can work for us or against us in the fight to keep our babies' heads round.

Now this solution may surprise you. We often think that the key to avoiding head flattening is to avoid pressure on the skull as much as possible. *Maintaining or regaining a round head requires more than alleviating or avoiding pressure on your baby's head. It requires strategically applying pressures to help shape the skull.* Now that we've uncovered the truth about what causes head flattening and the key ingredient in the solution, we're really heading in the right direction for a Fix.

Within this book, we'll look at many strategies, tools and tips for strategically applying pressures to help shape your baby's skull. I'll divide these into two different categories – **Proactive Positioning** and **repositioning**.

Maybe you've been offered no information about how your baby's positioning throughout every day and night affects head shape (and development). Or maybe you were merely told to turn your baby's head different directions during sleep and to do Tummy Time. It's time that every parent hear the message about the importance of what I call **Proactive Positioning** – intentionally varying your baby's position throughout the day in order to help *prevent* head flattening in the first place. **Proactive Positioning** is the head flattening equivalent of eating a balanced diet to maintain your optimum health. **Proactive Positioning** can start the moment your baby is born (or the moment you put this book down).

You'll finish this book with a solid understanding of **Proactive Positioning** that includes baby's sleep time and awake time and spans all areas of baby care. You'll have a "toolbox" full of tips, tricks and strategies for preventing head flattening through positioning.

If your baby already shows signs of head flattening, you'll need a slightly different "toolbox" for strategically applying pressure through positioning. I like to describe **repositioning** as changing your baby's positioning and routines in order to provide different pressures on the skull in response to signs of flattening. **Repositioning** can start the moment you notice a flat spot forming and can slow, stop or reverse head flattening.

I've said it before and I'll say it a few more times before this book is through – the strategies that you use to prevent or manage Flat Head Syndrome also promote your baby's healthy motor, sensory and cognitive development and help give your baby the healthiest start possible. Putting the plan in this book into action will put you in the running for new parent of the year with any early childhood specialist you meet!

_____

# PART II.

# MY BABY'S HEAD IS ROUND - ISN'T IT?

_____

# CHAPTER 8.

## WEEKLY HEAD SHAPE CHECKS

---

When I ask parents when they first noticed their baby's head flattening, you know what kinds of responses I hear again and again?

"I didn't notice until the doctor pointed it out at her 4 month check up,"

"I thought maybe it looked a little flat in the back but I wasn't sure."

You spend so much of your time with this adorable new person in your life, how could you have not even noticed her head shape changing? Well, there's been a lot going on for you since this little one joined your family! You're busier than ever caring for an infant, navigating huge family adjustments, and trying to figure out how to remove various bodily fluids from clothing. Besides that, when you look at your baby, you're much more likely to gaze love-drunk into her eyes and make ridiculous cooing noises at her than to notice the shape of her cranium.

Those reasons are *totally understandable*. **But letting flat spots go undetected and/or unmanaged for a month or two until your child's next well-baby check-up allows them to worsen and loses valuable time to make the small changes needed to stop and reverse flattening.** So what's the secret to catching head flattening early? It's as easy as instituting a 3-step weekly head shape check and taking a few photos.

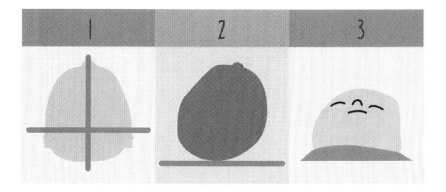

### Step 1 – Get a bird's eye view of your baby's head

Get directly above your little one's head. **Take a photo.** That way you can look carefully at it without baby wiggling and you'll be able to compare pictures from week to week for changes, which many parents have found tremendously helpful.

Divide the head into 4 quadrants by imagining 2 lines: one from nose to back of head and one from ear to ear (or from one ear to where the other should be). Ask yourself:

- Do the front two quadrants look symmetrical and equally full? What about the back two?
- Does the left half of your infant's head match the right in size, fullness and shape?
- Are the ears even?
- Does the back of baby's head look significantly less full and round than the front? (as in the illustration above)

### Step 2 – Look at how the head rests on a firm surface

When baby is lying on his back and you look at the top of his head, you'll be able to see several important features that can highlight flattening. Again, snap a photo to take a closer look and to save for future comparison. Ask yourself:

- Is one part of the back of baby's head not making as much contact with the floor as the other?
- Is baby's head tilted to one side or the other due to a flat spot? (as in the illustration above)
- Is there any bulging or slanting of the forehead to the left or right?

### Step 3 – View from the chin up

With baby still on his back, reposition yourself to get a clear view from his chin up. Snap your photo and closely examine it as you ask yourself:

- Does baby's forehead slope left or right? (as in the illustration above)
- Do baby's eyebrows look the same? Is his chin in the center? Are his lips aligned? Do his cheekbones appear even?

This head shape check isn't meant to be a substitute for physical examination by a medical professional if you have concerns about your baby. But, you are the person who is likely with your child the most and – *if you know what to look for – you can be the first person to notice flattening*. If keeping your baby's head round is important to you (and after reading the first section of this book, I hope it is), this easy head shape check will help you get there.

### Photography Tips:

- If your baby has thick hair, wet and slick the hair down to clearly reveal the shape of the head.
- Have an extra adult present – one of you to hold the baby and one to take the photos.

- Your baby's ears and nose will be important landmarks for photos – if they are obscured, have an adult point with finger(s) to the obscured landmark(s).

- If possible, keep the distance from the camera to the baby relatively consistent from week to week.

- Date the photos. A low-tech solution is to place a sticky note with the date on baby's shirt or the background in the photos.

**Baby Steps:**

Pick a day of the week and time that you consistently have another adult to help you take photos for a few moments. Get out your planner, open your calendar app or whip out some post-it notes for the fridge. Put a weekly head shape in writing each week for baby's first 6 months and begin this week!

# CHAPTER 9.

# A LOOK AT DIFFERENT HEAD SHAPES

Now that you're looking a bit more closely at your baby's head shape (and very likely the head shapes of other babies you see), let's take a look at the different ways babies can experience head flattening. What exactly am I talking about when I say Flat Head Syndrome?

Some babies experience flattening that makes their head look lopsided. This one-sided, asymmetrical flattening is called **Plagiocephaly**. Unfortunately, head flattening is a package deal – flattening of one area is usually accompanied by bulging or shifting in other areas of the head. In the case of Plagiocephaly, flattening on one side of the back of the head, often leads to that same side of the forehead pushing forward and the ear shifting forward. Because of this, the Plagiocephalic head shape is often described as a parallelogram. It's okay if you don't remember high school geometry and feel curious enough to Google 'parallelogram'!

To make matters a bit confusing, there are many terms used to describe Flat Head Syndrome. *Deformational Plagiocephaly* and *Positional Plagiocephaly* are sometimes used as umbrella terms to describe several different flattened head shapes. You probably haven't been getting much sleep since getting pregnant or welcoming a new baby into your home (I know I haven't), so for the sake of both of our sleep-deprived brains I'll keep things simple. In this book I'll use "Flat Head Syndrome" or "head flattening" to describe all of the head shapes described here and "Plagiocephaly" only to refer to asymmetrical flattening.

Other babies' heads get flat evenly, all the way across the back of the skull. Because this flattening is symmetric, it can be extra tough to spot. But if you look carefully at a baby with this head shape, called **Brachycephaly**, you'll probably notice some bulging or fullness of the forehead and/or widening of the skull, particularly noticeable just above the ears. It is also not uncommon to notice a high, raised area of the back of the skull just above the area of flattening. This is a very common head shape for babies who have primarily slept in baby gear like bouncy seats and infant car seat carriers. But, I'm getting ahead of myself!

Some babies really win the head shape lottery by having both broad flattening across the whole back of the skull and some asymmetrical flattening to boot. This is called **Brachycephaly with Plagiocephaly**.

While these first three head shapes are by far the most common, there's one more that I should mention. Some babies develop narrow and elongated heads, especially if they were premature and spent their early days in the NICU lying on their sides. Fortunately, most NICUs now have protocols for changing babies' positions as often as possible. Of course, some medical interventions won't allow for this, and head shape issues are far less important than a premature baby's overall health. The other major cause of this narrow and elongated head shape, called **Scaphocephaly** (also called Dolicephaly or Dolichocephaly), is womb positioning.

Unlike the first three head shapes we've looked at, this narrow and long head shape very rarely appears after the newborn period and can very closely resemble Craniosynostosis. For these reasons, extra care should be given to ensure an accurate diagnosis if you begin to notice significant narrowing or elongation of your baby's head after the first few weeks of life.

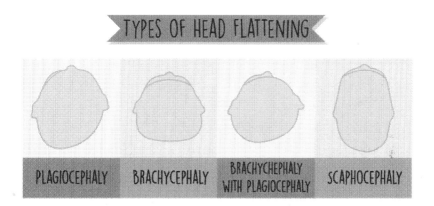

TYPES OF HEAD FLATTENING

PLAGIOCEPHALY | BRACHYCEPHALY | BRACHYCHEPHALY WITH PLAGIOCEPHALY | SCAPHOCEPHALY

# CHAPTER 10.

## PREFERRED POSITIONS AND TORTICOLLIS

---

There's a really important issue that we need to tackle before we move on in order to have a fuller understanding of Flat Head Syndrome. Babies grow all curled up and squished in the womb. When they make their debut in the world, it is VERY common for our little ones to have very subtle muscle tightness that can cause them to have *preferred positions.*[7,32]

Often, these muscle imbalances result in a preferred direction to turn the head (most often to the right), a slight head tilt toward one shoulder or a subtle curve of the spine and body toward one side.[12] As you can imagine, a preferred position means that baby spends more time with pressure on one part of the head, greatly increasing the risk of head flattening in that area. And just like subtle changes in head shape, many parents don't notice these imbalances until they create bigger problems.

Most of the time, the key to babies overcoming this very slight muscle tightness is plenty of time for movement. Through wiggling and kicking and reaching and turning the head, most babies naturally strengthen and stretch out of their preferred positions. We'll talk more in the next section about how something very simple that your baby likely does for hours every day can make these imbalances much worse. And of course, I'll share with you a collection of the absolute best tips for helping your baby work out of preferred positions.

## When Preferred Positions Persist

*Sometimes babies are born with or develop more significant neck tightness that greatly limits their neck movement and head position.* This is called Torticollis, which sounds like a scary medical word but is actually just Latin for "twisted neck". Torticollis results in a head that's tilted and/or rotated to one side due to muscle tightness. While there are many possible causes that can affect people at different ages, in this book I'll be referring to Torticollis of infancy. This includes both Congenital Muscular Torticollis (present at birth) and Positional Torticollis (acquired in infancy). The reason this neck issue deserves some attention in a book about head shape is the fact that *80-90% of babies with Torticollis wind up with some degree of Flat Head Syndrome.*[11]

What begins as an issue of the neck can very easily grow to be an issue of head shape, delayed milestones and of long-term developmental effects.

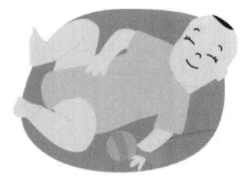

**Long-Term Difficulties in Babies With Unresolved Torticollis:**

- posture compensations when sitting and standing that often result in back muscle tightness and asymmetry of the spine
- decreased use of one arm for reaching, grasping, touch exploration, crawling, pulling to a stand, etc.
- resistance to Tummy Time and other positions requiring neck or upper body strength
- decreased visual and touch exploration of one side of baby's environment and his own body
- delayed gross motor skills such as rolling, crawling, pulling to a stand, walking8
- delayed fine motor skills such as grasping and using two hands together to handle objects

**Will this go away on its own?**

You might be wondering how you'll know whether your baby is showing signs of Torticollis that needs therapy or simply the common muscle asymmetries that typically resolve on their own with ample time for free movement. First, you should discuss all concerns with your child's physician. Second, from my experience:

A baby by 2 months of age…

- who shows preferred positions but is *able* to turn the head both directions on his own
- AND does not have a distinct and consistent head tilt (ear toward shoulder)
- AND shows no signs of head flattening

…will very likely work out of asymmetries by the 4 month well-baby check-up *if the family undertakes diligent **repositioning*** as described in Part Four of this book.

A baby by 2 months of age...

- who shows preferred positions
- AND does not appear *able* to turn the head in both directions
- AND/OR has a distinct and consistent head tilt (ear toward shoulder)
- AND shows signs of head flattening

...will benefit most from a comprehensive evaluation and recommendations from a skilled pediatric therapist.

A baby by 3 months of age...

- who continues to demonstrate preferred positions
- AND may or may not have head flattening

...will benefit most from a comprehensive evaluation and recommendations from a skilled pediatric therapist.

Torticollis can present in many ways affecting different muscles; *if your baby has been diagnosed with Torticollis, discuss the positioning strategies mentioned in this book with members of his care team.* You may be advised to avoid or modify certain positions or to emphasize others, based on which muscles are tight in your baby's neck and body.

**My doctor gave me a handout of stretches. Is this enough?**

Often, a physician who recognizes Torticollis will give parents a printed sheet of neck stretches to do at home. The vast majority of parents I've worked with get home, try a few stretches and stop. Why? Because their baby cries, they feel unsure that they're doing the stretches correctly, they are terrified of hurting their child and lack the support they need to feel comfortable with home therapy.

How well a family is able to implement Torticollis treatment at home is one of the biggest factors for how well a baby does in overcoming neck tightness.[21] If you don't feel equipped to provide treatment at home based on a worksheet, please speak up and request that your doctor refer your child to a therapist who can support your efforts. And please, don't rely on YouTube videos to instruct you in the medical care of your child's neck muscles! Remember that game of "Telephone" from elementary school? The more times a message is passed on, the more likely it is to be inaccurate. For your child's health, please seek out accurate, individualized stretching recommendations from a trained medical professional.

### What about Chiropractic Care and Alternative Therapies?

Many families are curious about the role of Chiropractic care and various forms of body work for the treatment of muscle tightness in their babies. For babies with Torticollis, I've seen wonderful results from these therapies in combination with Physical or Occupational Therapy. But I always recommend including therapy.

Why both? Because muscle tightness isn't just a body issue. It affects how a baby moves and plays. While a body worker addresses the spine and muscles around it and may use similar techniques to a pediatric therapist, the therapist works on the related movement and developmental effects of muscle tightness.

### Baby Steps:

Wherever you store photos of your little one (on your phone, computer, camera), take 3 minutes to quickly scroll through all the photos you can with one thing on your mind – your baby's head and body position. Notice if your little one's head is consistently turned chin toward one shoulder or tilted ear toward one shoulder (or both). Do you notice her body bending in one direction in a slight "C" shape? In my experience, a simple scroll through their photos is one of the most effective ways for parents to notice preferred positions in their sweet babes.

PART III.

---

# KEEP IT ROUND

---

# CHAPTER 11.

# A BALANCED POSITIONING DIET

---

Remember the Food Guide Pyramid of the 1990s? You probably colored one in elementary school and saw them on the sides of cereal boxes. The wide base of the pyramid was filled with grains and starches, fruits and vegetables. It represented the bulk of a healthy diet, or at least what we understood to be a healthy diet at the time. The top, or smallest portions of the pyramid, depicted fats, oils and sweets to be used sparingly.

I'm going to use the same pyramid concept to talk about *a balanced positioning diet for babies.* I imagine you're scratching your head at that one! Preventing Flat Head Syndrome is all about balancing the pressures on your baby's head – avoiding too much time in positions that put pressure on the same areas. To keep her head round and give your baby the best shot at being one of the 50% of babies who don't experience head flattening, you'll need to gain a clear understanding of how her positioning affects the pressures on her skull.

Imagine you knew nothing about nutrition. Nothing. No food guide pyramid, no diet books or health gurus on the nightly news had ever given you the information you needed to determine which foods are better for you than others. Your diet would likely be based on taste and convenience alone. What would you be eating? I would live off of Nutella and ice cream. It wouldn't be a good situation.

We need to understand different types of foods and have some guidance about how they affect our bodies in order to make wise choices for a balanced diet. In the exact same way, we need to understand the different positions our babies experience each day in order to provide balanced pressures on the head (and promote healthy development. Have I mentioned that these principles promote healthy development?).

Without a full understanding of and awareness of our babies' positioning, we tend to default toward an unbalanced "positioning diet" based on what's convenient, what's cute and what everyone else is doing. Why wouldn't we? If I could live off of Nutella and ice cream with no negative consequences, I most certainly would. But here's the thing, friends, *the alarming and growing rates of Flat Head Syndrome are a red flag (one of several that we're seeing in the world of child development) that there are negative consequences of our babies' unbalanced positioning diets.*

To help clarify our discussion of a healthy positioning diet for preventing Flat Head Syndrome, I'd like to share with you my Proactive Positioning Pyramid. Later, I'll share several Repositioning Pyramids that have been modified to emphasize positions that can slow, stop or reverse different types of head flattening. If your little one's head already shows signs of flattening, I know you're feeling the urge to skip ahead. But just as everyone needs a solid understanding of nutrition in order to change an out-of-balance diet, it will be tremendously important for you to have the firm foundation from this part of the book in order to best use the tools and strategies in the next part.

We'll discuss each position in detail, but let's start with a bird's-eye-view of the Proactive Positioning Pyramid.

# CHAPTER 12.

# THE PROACTIVE POSITIONING PYRAMID

Of all the ways I've talked to parents about how the positioning of their babies affects head shape, this super simple Pyramid illustration I made up has proven time and time again to be the most effective. It switches on a light bulb for parents and completely shifts the way they think about how their babies spend the day. Better yet, it *motivates* them to make the changes needed to give their babies the healthiest start possible. This is good news, because despite the fact that I'm cheering you on with Richard Simmons-level enthusiasm (but thankfully not with his wardrobe) to prevent and reverse Flat Head Syndrome, it's pretty hard to convey that encouragement through the pages of a book.

One hugely, massively important detail: the Proactive Positioning Pyramid is intended for babies with NO signs of head flattening and NO strong or persistent positional preferences (head turn, head tilt, body lean, etc.). In future chapters, we'll discuss ways to modify this Pyramid for babies with different types of head flattening or favored positions.

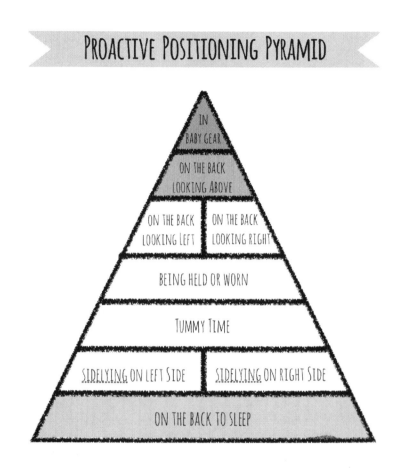

## PROACTIVE POSITIONING PYRAMID

IN BABY GEAR

ON THE BACK LOOKING ABOVE

ON THE BACK LOOKING LEFT | ON THE BACK LOOKING RIGHT

BEING HELD OR WORN

TUMMY TIME

SIDELYING ON LEFT SIDE | SIDELYING ON RIGHT SIDE

ON THE BACK TO SLEEP

You'll notice that the Pyramid doesn't offer "serving sizes" or specific time periods. Sometimes (often) we crave certainties as parents, but the Pyramid isn't meant to be rigid or prescriptive. It respects the fact that every baby is different, every day is different and you have to parent from your gut. The Proactive Positioning Pyramid is a general illustration meant to give you a framework for thinking about the pressures on your baby's head (and promoting her healthy development, right?).

You'll immediately notice that the wide base, the foundation, of the pyramid is the Back to Sleep position. Your little one will spend the majority of every 24 hour period snoozing while you spend the bulk of your time wishing you could get more sleep. Oh, the irony! Because of this fact, ***the priority of the whole rest of*** *the pyramid is to vary baby's position to minimize pressures across the back of the head and apply pressures to the sides of the head.*

Let's jump to the top of the pyramid and take a glance at those top two positions – in baby gear and on the back looking above. Since they mimic the pressures of the Back to Sleep position (and add some other risks that we'll chat about in upcoming chapters), they form the top of the pyramid. They are "to be used sparingly" – like Nutella and ice cream. Many, many babies with and without head flattening are spending the bulk of their days in these first three positions – on the back to sleep, in baby gear and on the back looking above (usually under an activity gym).[14] Of extra concern is the number who are sleeping in baby gear – but we'll tackle that topic soon enough.

Smack dab in the middle of the pyramid are 6 sections that are analogous to the fruits, veggies and protein of the Food Guide Pyramid – healthy, yummy goodness. Don't get too hung up on the sizes of the different sections. As long as you're equally balancing positions that put pressure on the right and left sides of the head and offering your baby regular, daily time in each of these positions, you're doing great. Different babies will tolerate these positions differently, and the amount of time spent in each will undoubtedly change through your little one's different ages and stages.

**Baby Steps:**

Take a quick moment to envision what your baby's Positioning Pyramid would look like right now. With your new understanding of the importance of offering baby a wide variety of positions to change pressures on the head, would you say your baby is enjoying a Balanced Positioning Diet?

If not, what is one single position that you could decrease your baby's time in to add balance?

What are one or two alternative positions that you could increase your baby's time in?

# CHAPTER 13.

# HEALTHY AND SAFE SLEEP POSITIONING

---

Your baby must be **safe**.

Safety trumps head shape every single time. We can agree on that, right? So while the Back to Sleep recommendations *do* increase your baby's risk of head flattening, I stand behind them. I encourage parents to learn all the recommendations for a safe sleep environment (which include much more than simply placing baby on her back to sleep) to reduce the risk of Sudden Infant Death Syndrome. These recommendations were put forth by the National Institute of Child Health and Human Development and are supported by the American Academy of Pediatrics.[24]

Are you one of the many parents surprised to know that sleeping in an infant swing, bouncy seat, napping chair and other baby gear increases your baby's SIDS risk and is specifically discouraged by the organizations I just mentioned? Even while awake, babies are at increased risk of getting less oxygen to the brain when they spend long periods in this type of baby seat.[3,23]

*Flat on the back to sleep is safest.*

So why does it seem like everyone you know is telling you that a Rock 'n Play is the golden ticket to sleepytime for you and your baby? Why are the most popular strollers the ones that allow your baby to snooze away in an infant car seat carrier for hours while you run errands or get your daily exercise?

Think back to when we talked about making positioning choices without fully understanding their effects on baby's health and development. Most parents simply don't know and so their decisions are based on what's convenient, what's cute and what everyone else is doing. Now, think back to the affirmations you stated earlier in this book. *You know more now than you did before and that will make you a better parent.*

If you're ready to break the habit of letting your baby sleep in baby gear but nervous about the transition to sleeping flat in a crib, bassinet or other firm, flat surface, I get it. Disrupting what's working to help your little one sleep can be terrifying. Maybe you're imagining all night crying spells and days with no naps. Here's where swaddling your infant can be one of your best tools. It provides calming sensory input to your baby and reduces the impact of the Startle Reflex normally seen in newborns. If you struggle with getting a solid swaddle with a thin blanket, there are tons of great "easy swaddles" available that allow you to snap, velcro or wrap your baby with ease. Be sure to stop swaddling when your baby begins rolling independently. I've shared more tips on helping your baby transition from sleeping in baby gear to sleeping flat on the back on the blog at CanDoKiddo.com (simply search for 'sleeping flat').

**Proactive Positioning For Sleep**

Let me guess – your baby doesn't sleep for as long at a time as you'd like. That's normal. It sure doesn't feel normal, does it? The silver lining to infant sleep patterns is that they allow frequent opportunities for influencing your baby's sleep position to change the pressures on her head.

There's one important caveat to Proactive Positioning for sleep. You really can't safely force a baby's head position for sleep. Sure, there are products available – pillows, hats and mattresses – that claim to prevent or reduce Flat Head Syndrome. But because they don't meet Safe to Sleep guidelines for SIDS reduction, *I do not recommend these products for sleeptime* (we will look in upcoming chapters at how these products might be helpful during awake times). So we're going to have to embrace the fact that all we can do is try to *influence* baby's head position for sleep. Your efforts to influence your little one's head position can make an impact, and every little bit of time with varying pressures on the head is progress! On to the strategies…

### Your Proactive Positioning Toolbox for Sleep

**Gently guide your baby's head to turn in a different direction (left or right) each time you place her down asleep.** If you find it hard to remember which direction you turned her the last time you put baby down, try keeping two sticky notes in the nursery ("right" and "left") and putting whichever one you did last on the wall, or try keeping a rubber band on one of your wrists or any other simple system you (and other caregivers) find works. This strategy tends to be most effective when you place baby down already asleep.

**Change which end of the crib you put your baby's head toward each day.** When falling asleep and upon waking, babies tend to turn toward the stimulation of the room and away from a solid wall. Your little one may also watch you as you walk out the door before falling asleep or turn toward the door in anticipation of you returning. You're kind of a big deal to your baby! If your baby sleeps in the room with you, she'll be more likely to turn toward you. By alternating which end of the crib you place baby's head toward (still on her back), you vary which side her head is most likely to turn toward as she falls asleep and wakes up.

**Place a mobile or other toy on one side of the crib.** Again, the idea here is that you're encouraging baby to turn her head a specific direction as she falls asleep as a way of influencing her head position during sleep. The safest sleep environment for reducing your baby's risk of SIDS is free of all stuffed animals, crib bumpers, blankets and toys. However, before baby can sit up and reach, you can attach toys securely to the crib rails higher up than she could roll into. This is important – be sure that you are either switching which end of the crib baby's head is at *or* switching the crib toy from one side to the other. The goal is to alternate baby's head position.

**Avoid mobiles that hang directly over baby's crib.** By now you very likely see how hanging a mobile or any other suspended toy or decoration directly over baby's crib would encourage her to maintain her head in a centered position as she falls asleep. Our goal is for baby to spend part of her sleeping time with the head turned each direction, so toys or nursery decor right over baby aren't going to be helpful.

**Consult your child's doctor.** Discuss with your child's doctor the risks/safety of allowing baby to sleep in a variety of positions while held, when closely supervised for naps or when on a parent's body. For children at lower risk of SIDS, some doctors will support this option for reducing the amount of sleep time spent flat on the back of the head. *Parents must make individual decisions about safe sleep for their babies (and assume all related risks) with full understanding of risks and benefits.*

# CHAPTER 14.

# INCONVENIENT TRUTHS ABOUT BABY GEAR

Sticking with our balanced diet analogy, have you ever been eating something totally melt-in-your-mouth delicious then flipped over the package to look at the nutrition facts only to have your jaw hit the floor? *Well, no wonder it's so good – it's nothing but butter and sugar!*

Well, friends, you may have a similar experience as we talk about some truths about baby gear. Once you know, you won't be able to unknow, and that infant swing might not look quite as appealing. I promise that this knowing is a vital part of *The Flat Head Fix*, and the truth you'll discover here will help you make wise and intentional choices about how you use baby gear. And – deep breaths – we won't throw the baby out with the bathwater (or the bouncy seat). You'll still be able to use the baby items you have in moderation while keeping your babe's head round and (say it with me) promoting healthy development.

There is a category of baby items I call "Baby Holding Devices." You may hear them referred to by child development specialists as "baby containers" or "baby buckets." You may hear them referred to by fellow parents as "life savers," "must-haves" or "essentials." Whatever you call them, they all support your baby in a semi-reclined, lounging, laid back position.

**Supportive Semi-Reclined Baby Holding Devices:**

- car seats and infant car seat carriers (including use outside of the car, as a stroller seat, etc.)
- bouncy seats
- rocking seats
- infant swings
- napping wedges
- lounge pillows

*This is not an exhaustive list – new variations of Baby Holding Devices hit the market all the time.

**Note that baby carriers that allow baby to be worn upright against a caregiver's body are not included in this list. These will be discussed in an upcoming section.

New and expectant parents get giddy registering for all these adorable pieces of baby gear that come highly recommended by fellow parents, magazines and websites. A house full of new baby gear is a sure sign that you're ready for your bundle of joy, right?

The problem is that parents don't usually realize the negative consequences of overusing Baby Holding Devices and aren't aware of what moderate use of baby gear looks like. The result? *Even when moved from device to device to device – from infant swing to car seat carrier to bouncy seat – babies are spending TOO MUCH TIME in the same position.* In fact, some studies suggest that the average baby may be spending 5 or more hours per day in various Baby Holding Devices.9

If you think back to our Proactive Positioning Pyramid, this position is in that small section at the tip-top – to be used sparingly. Let's talk about WHY time spent in baby gear should make up the smallest portion of your baby's day if keeping your baby's head round and promoting healthy development are your priorities.

**What Lounging In Baby Gear Does To Your Baby's Head**

*Most of the time that your sweet little one is lounging in an infant seat the greatest pressure is on the back of her head.* Remember, because babies spend so much time asleep with pressure across the back of the skull, this is a position and pressure we want to avoid as much as possible when baby is awake to avoid flattening.[18] Also, remember that sleeping in baby gear has safety risks for your precious little one and isn't recommended by doctors.

You might be thinking, "But it's so soft – that certainly won't make her head as flat as a firm mattress!" The fact that you're thinking about how pressures on the back of your baby's skull affect head shape is a huge step – nice work! However, a round head on a flat mattress is much easier to fully turn in either direction than a round head enveloped in a soft, rounded cushion, and therefore it's easier for a baby to independently change the pressures on her head while sleeping on a firm surface.20 For each additional hour of average daily time spent in baby gear in your baby's third and fourth months of life, her risk of Flat Head Syndrome as much as doubles!10

**How Time in Baby Gear Makes Preferred Positions Worse**

Recall the good news that given plenty of time free to move (like on a blanket on the floor), most babies stretch and strengthen out of preferred positions. But here's the bad news – when movement is restricted by soft, cushiony Baby Holding Devices that support baby in a slightly curled position (similar to the womb position), babies get less time to work out of their asymmetries.

The even worse news? Infants don't yet have the muscle strength and control to keep their bodies and heads upright against gravity. When baby is placed in a semi-reclined position, gravity very often pulls her into those asymmetric preferred positions we talked about. This can make those minor muscle asymmetries much worse and longer-lasting. Because preferred positions result in baby spending more time with pressure on one part of the head, *baby gear that worsens preferred positions increases your baby's risk of developing Flat Head Syndrome.*

**What your baby is NOT doing in a Baby Holding Device**

To make matters even worse, by spending too much time in baby gear, our little ones are living at the top of the Positioning Pyramid, missing critical time in a variety of positions that prevent head flattening *and* promote healthy development. They miss opportunities to turn their heads through their necks' full range of motion, to respond to information from their senses about the world around them and to fully experience the full range of movements and sensations of their bodies.[29]

*Babies with high use of baby holding devices score lower on infant motor development tests than babies who don't spend as much time in equipment.*[1] As parents, we're blasted with information about reading and speaking to your baby for language development and playing music for brain development. But somehow the message isn't getting out that movement and play unrestricted by baby gear is important for infant wellness and development. Now you know!

"Oh, wait a second," you're thinking, "if you're suggesting I stop using these devices that give me sanity as a new parent, I'll just stop reading now!" Fear not, we're not going to talk about trashing your baby gear, merely about how to change your baby gear habits to reduce the negative impacts on your child's head shape and development.

# CHAPTER 15.

# MODERATE AND INTENTIONAL BABY GEAR USE

---

If you now want to kick your baby gear to the curb, I certainly won't stop you. But for many families, bouncy seats, swings and infant car seat carriers used outside of the car feel like non-negotiable keys to surviving life with a new baby. I fully recognize that I might risk my life trying to pry a Rock 'n Play out of a new mom's fingers. Instead, I suggest that we explore some ways to be more moderate and intentional in how we use Baby Holding Devices.

*In order to keep time in Baby Gear in moderation and at the top of the Proactive Positioning Pyramid, I strongly advise new parents to limit baby's time to an average of two hours per day or less supported in a semi-reclined position in equipment.* This includes time in the car seat for travel.

When asked to total up the number of hours their baby spends on average per day in Baby Holding Devices, most parents I've worked with (whose babies have Flat Head Syndrome) come up with a number between 3 and 5 hours per day. For babies who regularly sleep in baby gear, this number easily increases to 10 or more hours per day.

Keeping in mind that this whole category of Baby Holding Devices holds baby in effectively the same position, let's look at a very normal morning outing for a new parent. Baby might spend 15 minutes in the bouncy seat while Mommy gets dressed for an errand, 15 minutes riding to the grocery store, 30 minutes still in the car seat carrier at the store, plus the ride home, 15 minutes in the swing while Mommy unloads groceries and an extra 30 minutes in the swing because baby fell asleep there. This one errand and nap would put baby at that recommended daily max of 2 hours. Not a huge deal if that was the full extent of baby's time in baby gear for the day. But if we're being realistic, for the majority of babies it's not.

So how can you break your dependency on Baby Holding Devices and bring your little one's Proactive Positioning Pyramid more into balance?

### Tips for Reducing Baby's Time in Baby Gear

- Use a sling, wrap or soft structured carrier to wear baby on errands (more in Chapter 20).

- Use a stroller with a bassinet attachment or seat that reclines flat instead of using your infant car seat carrier as the seat (more in Chapter 17).

- Place baby on a blanket on the floor to play and move with close supervision while you complete daily tasks at home (more in Chapters 18, 19 & 21).

- Move a sleepy or sleeping baby to a firm, flat sleep surface as soon as you can (obviously not while driving in the car).

- If a fussy baby, family travel or other circumstances result in extra time in baby gear one day, aim for less than 2 hours total time on the following few days.

- As much as possible, keep your car seat carrier in the car. Allow baby to spend time in other positions when you reach your destination – hold baby while waiting for your food at a restaurant, put a soft blanket on the ground at the park for baby while older siblings play nearby, let baby enjoy the different positions described in this book in a parked stroller with bassinet attachment or with the seat reclined flat.

Next, let's look at how to be proactive in our positioning of baby in baby gear when we DO choose to use it.

# CHAPTER 16.

# PROACTIVE POSITIONING IN BABY GEAR

---

For those times that you do choose to use baby gear, all hope is not lost. There are some strategies you can use to reduce the impacts on your baby's head shape. The key is knowing about them. So let's dive in!

**Good Posture for Babies**

Sometimes as parents, we have blinders on to what our own kids look like in baby gear. Our eyes are drawn to their sweet little eyes and chubby fingers, failing to see that they're often in really wonky positions. Sometimes I feel like the Baby Posture Police and have to fight the urge to straighten up strangers' babies who I see flopped over, curled up and ultimately squished in their car seat carriers. It's a job hazard, I suppose!

What's the big deal? Aside from the fact that these positions can restrict your little one's airway[2] (NOT a good thing!), they limit baby's ability to move and often reflect those preferred positions we've talked about, resulting in more pressure on one part of baby's head.

The simple fix? When you put baby in baby gear, take a few extra seconds to position her upright with shoulders directly in line with hips, chin away from chest, and ears away from shoulders. You can use rolled washcloths or receiving blankets to help support baby in a good posture but *do not add these props to a car seat when it's used in the car, which can reduce the safety of the car seat.*

Remember that for a baby with no signs of head flattening and no strong, persistent preferred positions, your Proactive Positioning goal is to encourage positions that reduce pressure on the back of the skull AND apply pressure to the sides of the head to combat the effects of sleeping on the back. Try these strategies to encourage your baby to look both directions and change the pressures on the head often while in baby gear.

### Your Proactive Positioning Toolbox for Baby Gear

**Intentionally position toys away from the middle of baby gear** (especially for toys with a toy bar or mobile). Alternate which side of baby gear you position toys on to promote head turning each direction. The ability to do this in a stroller bassinet or reclined flat stroller seat is a huge reason I recommend these seating options instead of an infant car seat carrier as stroller seat (more in Chapter 17).

**Remove mobiles or toys that encourage baby to keep head centered in baby gear.**

**Change the position of baby gear in the room.** Quite often, we don't even notice that baby consistently looks one direction in a swing or seat because "the action" of the room is on a particular side of her. Turn your gear regularly to encourage lots of different head positions.

**Gently turn a very young infant's head to look each direction.** Older, more active babies often hold positions for shorter durations but you may find that your newborn will continue to look the direction turned for several minutes.

**Use a stroller bassinet attachment or reclined flat stroller**

**seat** to help baby to have awake time in a variety of positions (Tummy Time, sidelying each side and on the back looking to each side) when the stroller is parked.

**Check and change baby's position in baby gear close to every 15 minutes** to help your baby resume that upright position I described. This is also a great time to get baby out for some playtime, sleeping time flat on the back or cuddle time worn or held. By getting into this habit, many parents find that they have an increased awareness of how long their baby actually spends in baby gear and that their dependence on that gear decreases as they realize that their baby can be happy in many other positions.

**Baby Steps:**

For the next few days, try to observe how much total time your little one is spending supported in a semi-reclined position in baby gear (use a timer app, notes on a scrap of paper, keep a running tally in your head or whatever solution works for you). Ask other caregivers to join you in monitoring your little one's time in gear. Raising your awareness of how time in all these different pieces of equipment adds up can be a huge wake-up call for parents and help motivate them to make small changes in how their baby is positioned throughout the day.

# CHAPTER 17.

# WHEN BABY'S IN A STROLLER

The popularity and perceived convenience of car seat travel system strollers have resulted in babies spending far more time in baby gear. Times that they would have been carried, worn or laid flat in a bassinet or pram-style stroller have been replaced by the semi-reclined position that exacerbates muscle asymmetries and limits freedom of movement, including head turning.

Instead of relying on a car seat as an infant positioner out of the car, I recommend parents use a stroller that allows them to lay their babies flat until they can sit upright with just a little support. While babywearing or carrying your little one are better options (and therefore are lower and larger on the Proactive Positioning Pyramid), they aren't always practical or feasible.

**Why flat on the back is better than semi-reclined?**

When flat on the back, baby isn't supported in a fixed position. She has greater freedom of movement of her arms, legs and head. In fact, strategically placing toys on the sides of the stroller can further encourage head turning and can be a valuable piece of Proactive Positioning. Instead of adding to your baby's time in the semi-reclined position of Baby Holding Devices, your stroller can move your little one down the Proactive Positioning Pyramid to the more beneficial "on the back with toys to the side" position.

Lying flat is also less likely to worsen any existing positional preferences because gravity isn't pulling your little one into asymmetrical body postures.

And finally, a stroller that reclines flat can allow baby to have awake time in a variety of positions when not in motion. While you enjoy a meal at a restaurant or playtime at the park with an older sibling, baby can be placed in sidelying or Tummy Time positions on the flat surface of the stroller.

**Check your stroller's seat recline**

You might be surprised to find that many strollers on the market today at all price points have the feature of a full seat recline (or within 15 degrees of flat). Even if you already own a car seat travel system stroller, check the seat recline to see if laying baby flat is an option for you. If you have the available resources, you might also consider a bassinet or pram-style stroller. It's a short-lived purchase but a far better investment in your baby's development than adding a Snap 'n Go or other frame-style stroller to your baby gear collection.

# CHAPTER 18.

## SIDELYING

As parents we hear *so much* about Back to Sleep and Tummy Time. In fact, they're often the only two positions we receive any guidance on! But our babies are not flat like pieces of paper to be flipped exclusively front to back and back to front. And our whole goal with *The Flat Head Fix* is to avoid their heads getting or staying flat. Because we're trying to overcome all the time that our babies are spending in the Back to Sleep position with pressure on the back of the head, I'd like to share a little-talked-about position that's a very powerful tool in fighting flat heads – sidelying.

Most parents aren't familiar with this term, and I certainly know my computer's spell-check isn't! Sidelying is just as simple as it sounds – laying baby on his side while awake. Babies tend to tolerate the supportive sidelying position very well in part because it requires less muscle effort than Tummy Time. Therapists and child development nerds like me love sidelying because it helps baby bring hands together, balance the strength of the back and belly muscles, experiment with partial-rolling (both intentionally and unintentionally), and it gives unique sensory information to the movement (vestibular) and pressure/stretch (proprioceptive) senses about body position.

**Your Proactive Positioning Toolbox for Sidelying**

**To prevent Flat Head Syndrome, be sure your baby receives equal time in both right and left sidelying positions.**

**Give your baby an object, book or toy in sidelying** to look at, touch or put in the mouth.

**Prop baby in sidelying.** If you find that your baby rolls easily out of sidelying, try propping her with a rolled towel or blanket behind her back (I find it's more stable if you tuck it under baby's play blanket) or use a 1 lb. bag of dried rice or beans. Once your baby is intentionally rolling, these props won't likely keep your little one in place, but they work very well in the first months of life.

**Sidelying as a break from Tummy Time.** Here's a trick I use very often in my work with babies. When your little one begins fussing in Tummy Time and is ready for a break, simply roll her to sidelying for a few minutes of play. Very often, she'll tolerate another minute (or two or three) of belly-down play after a break. Helping your baby feel the sensation of rolling into and out of the Tummy Time position is great sensory input and tends to improve Tummy Time tolerance compared to placing baby directly on a surface belly-down.

**Carry your baby in the sidelying position.** Carrying your baby in the sidelying position is a great way to stretch the muscles of your little one's neck and provide pressure on the side of baby's head. Position baby with her back against your chest or belly. Give her good support with one of your arms under her body (hand on the side of her ribcage) and one of your arms or hands under her head. Check to see that you're providing support on the side of baby's head near the ear instead of on her jaw.

**Sidelying on your lap.** Newborns fit perfectly in the sidelying position on your thighs with feet toward your belly and head toward your knees. Use a thin blanket to pad your knees, if needed.

**Sidelying with family on a couch or chair.** The crack between couch cushions covered with a blanket makes a great spot for baby to enjoy awake sidelying with close supervision. You can also prop baby in sidelying using the back or arms of a couch or upholstered chair with close supervision. Never leave baby unattended on a raised surface.

**Sidelying in a flat stroller.** One of several reasons that I recommend parents use a stroller that reclines flat or a bassinet-style stroller is that when you're not rolling along, you can vary your baby's position (unlike an infant car seat carrier used as a stroller seat). When eating at a restaurant, at the park with older siblings or on other outings place baby in sidelying to look at a toy or book. If you're not ready to stop using the car seat carrier as stroller seat completely, you might consider decreasing your baby's time in the car seat by moving her to the flat stroller seat for different positioning when you've arrived at your destination.

# CHAPTER 19.

# TUMMY TIME

---

If you're like most new parents, you've had questions about Tummy Time. Is it safe? Is it mean? What if baby cries? How long should baby do Tummy Time each day? How important is it really?

Let's clear up some of the confusion and equip you with Tummy Time goals, tips and tools.

## Tummy Time is about more than neck strength

In the belly-down position when an infant isn't actively lifting the head and rests with cheek down, *Tummy Time provides excellent stretching to the neck and the chest* and can help babies work out of minor muscle tightness and asymmetries. Tummy Time is also great for the sensory development that's essential for rolling, crawling, standing and all the other milestones you're looking forward to!

## Neck Strength is about More Than Neck Strength

Guess where the muscles of the neck attach? On the bones of baby's skull. And that means that neck muscles can have an impact on head shape. Strong, evenly developed neck muscles can help hold skull bones in place, while any neck tightness or imbalanced muscle strength can create asymmetrical pulls on bones and further increase your baby's risk of head

## Tummy Time Goals

30 minutes per day by the end of month 1
60 minutes per day by the end of month 2
90 minutes per day by the end of month 3

These goals are an average, so if a fussy baby day or family travel makes Tummy Time tricky, just aim for more Tummy Time over the next few days.

## Tips for Reaching Tummy Time Goals

These goals may sound high, but remember that they are broken up into many, many periods of daily Tummy Time for itty bitty babies. For example, if your newborn only tolerates the belly-down position for 1-2 minutes, aim to put baby in this position 15-30 times each day in the first month. Still sound like a lot? Let's look at a few of my biggest recommendations to families who are struggling to squeeze in enough Tummy Time.

**Make Tummy Time a part of your daily routines.** You're busy enough caring for an infant, let's not make Tummy Time an *extra* 30, 60 or 90 minute task to complete each day. Instead, find simple ways to add Tummy Time to the daily care and activities you're already doing for your little one. Carry your baby from the car to the house in Tummy Time on your forearm. Place baby in Tummy Time for a minute or two on the changing table while you get diaper change supplies ready or while you let her bottom air dry from being wiped (this habit is also great for preventing diaper rash). Roll baby into Tummy Time while you apply lotion after bathtime. Let baby enjoy Tummy Time on your lap as you visit with family or friends or sit in a doctor's office waiting room (if you haven't yet had your baby, consider yourself warned – there will be a lot of medical appointments for both of you in the first few months).

**Make Tummy Time a position for play.** Novelty will be one of your biggest tools for increasing your baby's Tummy Time. By incorporating creative, new sensory experiences in baby's playtime (like those in my book, *Begin With A Blanket* – available on Amazon), you capture her interest and help make Tummy Time enjoyable.

Do your best to give baby as much Tummy Time as possible. There's no max limit to how much baby can do in a day if he's happy in the belly-down position. BUT, *if you have a baby that for whatever reason is really miserable in Tummy Time, remember that there are several other really valuable positions for preventing Flat Head Syndrome.* Keep working on short, frequent periods of Tummy Time, but also increase your baby's time in the other positions in the middle of the Proactive Positioning Pyramid.

### Tummy Time Hints

- begin in the first week of life for healthy, full term infants*

- try Tummy Time on a parent or caregiver's body: on the lap, on the chest, carried on the forearm

- get face to face with your baby in Tummy Time

- slowly roll baby into and out of the Tummy Time position instead of placing directly belly-down

- allow baby to grunt, squawk and whine a bit; end Tummy Time only when baby is truly distressed

- take Tummy Time outside on a blanket or on your lap (weather permitting)

- pause for a few moments of Tummy Time in new places on errands – take 5 minutes to sit on a bench and let baby enjoy the sights belly-down on your lap (or pack a soft blanket on outings for Tummy Time on the floor or ground)

- enlist the help of a friend – an older sibling, family member or family pet can give baby lots of motivation to lift his head in Tummy Time

- place your hand or a 1 lb. bag of dried rice or beans on baby's low back/bottom in Tummy Time to help anchor her hips

- try Tummy Time over a Boppy pillow (nursing pillow) or lift baby's chest on a rolled towel or blanket

- help position a young infant's arms under her – elbows tucked under shoulders

- pat baby's back, sing, make faces – let baby know you're near

- position toys to match your baby's vision and head lifting abilities – keep toys close and low (or under baby's face if elevated on a Boppy or rolled blanket) or slightly to the side in the first two months and gradually move them further and higher as baby is able to lift and hold the head

- use accordion-style books or toys spread around baby to encourage head turning in Tummy Time

*Unless there are complications, there is no need to wait until baby's umbilical stump falls off to initiate Tummy Time. Typically, the newborn Tummy Time position is curled with knees and arms underneath, lifting the low belly off the surface.

**Your Proactive Positioning Toolbox for Tummy Time**

**Alternate which cheek is down.** In earliest weeks of Tummy Time help baby spend equal time with each cheek down. This cheek-down time is one of the *only* positions that applies pressure to the front-sides of your baby's head (near the temples) and is very, very valuable for combatting Flat Head Syndrome. You'll see in upcoming sections how important it can be for helping reshape baby's head if flattening has already started.

# CHAPTER 20.

# WEARING AND HOLDING YOUR BABY

---

### Babywearing

Do you see new parents wearing their babies in trendy carriers and assume that they're "crunchy?" You know the type – probably eat only organic foods grown in their own garden, drive hybrids only when their bicycles are in the shop, make their own clothing from hemp and free-range Alpaca fleece.

Please don't let babywearing stereotypes stop you from trying a wrap, sling or carrier another single day! Babywearing is for everyone and has been a primary means of transporting our adorable offspring throughout human history – long before "organic" and "free range" were even terms! You might be very surprised at how comfortable, convenient and sweet it is to have your little one snuggled up against you. And you'll definitely be relieved to know that wearing your baby is a fantastic position for reducing his risk of Flat Head Syndrome.

If, since starting this book, you're beginning to see that your baby's Positioning Pyramid is top-heavy from too much time in Baby Holding Devices, try wearing your baby as an alternative to using infant car seat carriers and travel system strollers when on outings with baby.

Maybe you're like the dozens of people who have asked, "is that comfortable?" when they see me wearing my baby. YES! There are many different styles of carriers, wraps and slings that can make babywearing very comfortable for most people and most babies. I comfortably wore my baby up to 25 pounds (and up to 20 weeks pregnant with his younger sibling)! There are many local and online babywearing groups that can help you choose and find the right carrier for you and your little one.

Perhaps you're thinking that all that wrapping of long stretchy fabric is a hassle. Again, there are many options available. If wrapping isn't your thing, find a carrier that you quickly slip baby into for use on errands.

The support of being worn allows an awake baby to work on the strength and motor control to hold his head up and turn toward sounds or sights in his environment. Even when a baby's head is supported against the wearer's chest (similar to that cheek down position in Tummy Time we talked about), pressure is eliminated on the back of the head, light pressure is applied to the front-sides of the head and the neck muscles are stretched.

### Your Babywearing Proactive Positioning Toolbox

**Support baby in an upright posture.** Because babywearing holds baby upright against gravity, it *can* pull baby into a preferred position just like Baby Holding Devices. Just as with baby gear, check your baby's posture and ensure that your carrier is snug enough to give your little one the support to remain upright.

**Alternate which of baby's cheeks is against you or which way your baby most often looks when worn** to promote equal head turning and equal neck stretching. You can do this gently with your hands for very young babies. For older babies, attaching a teething pad or teething toy to one side or one strap of the carrier is a great way to promote head turning. Be sure to move these items from side to side periodically.

**Support baby's legs.** Babywearing wraps, slings and carriers should support the back of baby's thighs fully to protect his yet underdeveloped hip joints (preventing legs dangling from the hips). For safety as well as developmental and physical reasons, it is generally recommended that babies be worn facing toward a parent's chest for the first 6 months or until baby shows great interest in turning to see the world.

## Carrying and Holding Your Baby

Seems funny to be reading tips for holding your baby, doesn't it? The truth is, we easily fall into habits and patterns very early on in parenting. How you most frequently carry your baby is a *big one*. An important part of Proactive Positioning is bringing some awareness to the ways you hold and carry your little bundle of joy and making tweaks if needed to break those habits.

### Your Proactive Positioning Toolbox For Carrying & Holding

**Switch sides.** Alternate which arm (and later, which hip) you carry your baby on.

**Change baby's positions.** Hold baby in a Tummy Time position on your forearm(s), in a sidelying position, upright on each of your shoulders, forward-facing while cradled against your chest, on her back in each of your arms, supported fully by both of your hands in a seated position with chin supported, and more! By thinking more intentionally about your baby's positioning, you can get really creative and have fun with holding and carrying your baby in many different ways. Of course, safety is the top priority, and you'll always want to make sure baby's head is fully supported until she gains head control.

# CHAPTER 21.

## PLAYTIME ON THE BACK

---

I have to preface this and the following chapter by stressing how much I *love* activity gyms for babies. They offer wonderful opportunities for floortime play – time unrestricted by Baby Holding Devices, time to stretch and strengthen out of the fetal position and any preferred positions, opportunities to visually explore new things, reach, kick….oh, I could go on all day!

But here's the one thing I don't love about activity gyms – they can contribute to head flattening. Because it places similar pressures on your baby's head as sleeping on the back, playing on the back with toys suspended directly over your baby should be used sparingly as a daily position for your baby.

This position does have some great benefits, so it's not to be avoided completely. It's a great way for your little one to work on batting with the arms to hit toys, reaching and eventually grasping. It allows your little one to stretch and strengthen the muscles of his belly and legs as he extends and kicks his legs. *This position is much more developmentally beneficial than parking your little one in a Baby Holding Device but should be used in moderation to avoid contributing to head flattening.*

Don't despair, there's a really simple trick you can use to avoid this and make your baby's activity gym an ideal play spot. What's the secret?

**Your Proactive Positioning Toolbox For Play on the Back**

**Hang toys from the sides of your baby's activity gym instead of directly overhead.**

**Avoid activity gyms that have a moving and/or musical mobile in the center or that don't allow you to reposition toys.**

**Place toys beside your baby when she's playing on a blanket on the floor without an activity gym.** Toys with a few inches or more of height are perfect for this purpose so that they're easily seen by your little one. Propped books, mirrors, stuffed animals and balls are great toys to try.

CHAPTER 22.

# SIMPLE TWEAKS TO YOUR DAILY BABY CARE

---

Having a new baby means you feel busier than you've ever been, yet somehow you can't seem to get much done. How did it get to be 5:00 p.m. and you're still wearing pajamas and have unbrushed teeth? Oh, I've been there, too! Luckily, all this Proactive Positioning really doesn't require much more of your time; all it demands is your awareness and your willingness to make small changes. Let's look at some super easy tweaks you can make to your daily routines with baby that can make a big impact on her head shape.

### Diaper Changes

While baby lies on her back getting a fresh diaper (how can someone so small make so much waste?), you can encourage her to turn her head in different directions with just a few simple strategies. These will place diaper changes into the "On the back looking left/right" section of the Proactive Positioning Pyramid and reduce the time your baby spends with pressure flat on the back of the head.

Unless you've strategically placed toys, mobiles or artwork near your changing table, your baby is most likely to turn to look at you or other caregivers during diaper changes. *Most people find that there is a side that is easier to change a diaper on, which can set baby up to look in the same direction at each diaper change.* In the early months, with ten or more diaper changes a day each taking several minutes, that time can easily add up to an extra 30 minutes a day of your baby looking the same direction.

### Your Proactive Positioning Toolbox for Diaper Changes

**Switch the direction you lay your baby on the changing table.** If you're able to coordinate diaper changes with baby facing the other end of the table (i.e. alternate which is the head and foot sides of the table), alternating positions will change the direction baby is most likely to turn and encourage equal time on each side of the back of the head. However, make sure for sanitation purposes that your baby's head is being placed on a clean surface. This may mean that you alternate directions every few days after you wash or rotate the changing pad or cover.

**Strategically place and move toys.** Does changing a diaper with your non-dominant hand while suffering sleep deprivation max out your brain capacity? Don't worry, here's an alternative strategy. A few simple black and white pictures taped to the wall next to the changing table or a high-contrast toy placed on one side of the changing pad will encourage your little one to turn her head while being changed. If your changing table has rails, alternate which side you place toys or pictures on every few days. If you are only able to place toys or pictures on one side of the table, just remove them every few days instead and encourage baby to turn to face you to alternate head position.

### Feeding

You may not ever think about your baby's head positioning when feeding, but something so regular and routine in her life can definitely impact her head shape – for better or for worse. Let's make sure it's for better with a few proactive steps you can take to make sure feeding positioning isn't putting your baby at risk for head flattening.

## Your Proactive Positioning Toolbox for Feeding

**Be aware of breastfeeding positioning**. Most women naturally alternate sides when breastfeeding, which gives baby different pressures on the head. *In the rare case that you are only able to feed from one breast, alternate feeding positions such as the football hold and the cradle hold so that baby gets pressure on both sides of the head to help prevent flattening.* Consult with a Lactation Consultant or local breastfeeding support group to learn more about different positions.

**Alternate which arm you hold baby in for bottle feeding**. Exclusive bottle feeding is a significant risk factor for head flattening.7 This may be true because very often caregivers fall into habitual positions of feeding. One very common feeding position, bottle feeding with baby's head cradled in the crook of one arm while baby looks lovingly up at you, tends to place pressure on the side of baby's head closest to you. By alternating which arm you hold baby in, you alternate the pressures on the sides of her head and help reduce her risk of flattening. How easy is that?

# CHAPTER 23.

# SITTING - IS YOUR BABY READY?

---

After a few weeks of wobbling and a some inevitable head bonks, you'll celebrate the huge milestone of your baby sitting up. Suddenly, your squishy little infant is starting to look like a big baby. Don't blink – you'll be sending her off to Kindergarten if you do!

Sitting is a huge milestone for your baby's development and for her head shape. Once your baby can independently move into and out of sitting, she'll *likely* spend far less time with pressure across the back of the skull – a win for reducing the risk of Flat Head Syndrome! But, in order for this to be true, you must give her adequate opportunities to sit. *Far too many parents unknowingly prolong the period of increased risk of head flattening by continuing daily use of infant swings, bouncy seats, car seat carriers (outside the car) and other Baby Holding Devices after their baby reaches the milestone of sitting.*

Once your baby can sit, let her:

- sit in shopping carts on errands
- use a stroller with an upright seat
- sit on the floor for playtimes

- use a high chair with a fully upright seat (this is also better positioning for eating than semi-reclined chairs).

**Helping Your Baby Sit: Is He Ready Yet?**

It's important to wait until babies are showing signs of readiness for sitting before we begin to "sit them" or use baby seats. Propped in sitting before he's ready, a baby isn't able to support himself against gravity and is pulled into those preferred positions we've talked about. Even a baby with no positional preferences will be pulled by gravity into an unhelpful position with back rounded, pelvis tilted back, shoulders hunched and possibly an asymmetrical spine or neck position. It might be a cute look for monthly photos, but this type of early sitting on a regular basis doesn't help your baby achieve independent sitting any sooner and isn't good for his little body.

A better way to support a baby who isn't yet showing signs of readiness for sitting is to sit him in your lap, supporting his ribcage with your hands. Hold him as high up as you need in order for baby to show steady head control and the ability to freely move both arms. Gradually, as baby gains more head and trunk control over weeks and months, you can move your hands lower on the ribcage and eventually to the hips.

In general, I don't see baby seats as important pieces of baby gear. By the time a baby is showing readiness for sitting, the milestone of independent sitting is usually only a few weeks away, making baby seats (when used properly) very short-lived purchases. If you do choose to use a baby seat once your baby shows signs of readiness, I recommend limiting use to an average of 30 minutes or less per day. This is because these devices tend to support babies in a way that doesn't promote the skills needed for independent sitting. Time in baby seats also limits the time available for other positions that more effectively fight Flat Head Syndrome and promote healthy development. However, modified recommendations for using baby seats for babies with one specific type of head flattening are made in Chapter 27, so stay tuned!

**Signs of readiness for sitting:**

- baby is sitting with a tall, straight spine and steady head control in supported sitting
- baby is beginning to try to move into and out of hands and knees position
- baby is starting to reach arms out to the front or sides to protect against a fall in sitting

PART IV.

_____

# ROUND IT BACK OUT

_____

# CHAPTER 24.

# IS FLAT HEAD SYNDROME REALLY REVERSIBLE?

If the reality is that your baby's head is flattening, your first reaction might be to feel worried. Or discouraged. Or defensive. Or guilty. *These are all very normal and very common reactions.* Especially that last one. In fact, let's take a moment to repeat those words of reassurance from the beginning of this book:

*I have always tried to do what's best for my child to the best of my knowledge. When I know more than I did before, it helps me be a better parent.*

Feel free to print those out and tape them to your bathroom mirror if you're really battling guilt. There's great news, though! There are proven **repositioning** methods for slowing, stopping and even reversing Flat Head Syndrome.

I share this great news with fair warning: sometimes diligent **repositioning** requires effort. The strategies I've compiled are not rocket science or complicated, but they do require extra attention and some new habits. Just like there's no easy button for having a baby, there isn't an effortless fix for Flat Head Syndrome. But if you're willing to put the effort in and keep your focus on the long-term goal of giving your baby the healthiest start possible, you can achieve great results.

Do the methods in *The Flat Head Syndrome Fix* guarantee that your baby's head will be perfectly round or that a helmet won't be recommended for your child? No. In some cases, even with diligent **repositioning**, Flat Head Syndrome is persistent and severe enough to warrant a conversation about using a helmet. In Chapter 31, I'll share valuable tips for facing that decision with confidence.

**How Does Repositioning Work?**

In order to understand repositioning, it's helpful to understand how helmets designed to treat Flat Head Syndrome work. Baby helmets give space around the areas of skull flattening while placing pressure (or "holding") more rounded areas of the head. In much the same way, we can be strategic in **repositioning** our babies during sleep time and awake time in order to reduce or eliminate pressure on areas of flattening and focus pressure on areas of roundness. Increasing pressure to the rounded or bulging areas of a baby's skull encourages the head to grow into areas of flatness in the same way that a helmet would. *Diligent repositioning efforts, especially when started early, can effectively reshape or remold a baby's head, and some studies suggest that they can be as effective as helmets for the treatment of Plagiocephaly.*

How will you know that your repositioning efforts are paying off? I'd love to share some important tools for tracking your baby's changing head shape over time.

CHAPTER 25.

# ESTABLISH A BASELINE AND DOCUMENT CHANGE

Remember those weekly head shape checks from Chapter 8? *If you notice your baby developing a flat spot, it's important to keep doing those head shape checks and taking weekly photos.*

**Why?**

As you commit to the **repositioning** strategies of *The Flat Head Syndrome Fix,* you'll want to know whether your baby's head is getting less flat, more flat or staying the same as a result of your efforts.

Taking weekly photos throughout a period of diligent **repositioning** has allowed many parents to feel much more confident when faced with the question of whether or not to pursue a helmet. Additionally, some insurance companies require documentation that several months of repositioning have been ineffective in correcting head shape in order to pay for helmets.

*Seeing how your baby's head shape has changed over time will be an important tool for you and your baby's care team to effectively determine "next steps" in the weeks and months ahead.*

**5 Photos To Take Each Week**

Once a week, taking 5 photos of your little one will give you an incredibly useful timeline of head shape changes.
1. Bird's eye view
2. Right profile (right side of head)
3. Left profile (left side of head)
4. From the chin up with back of head on a firm surface
5. From the top with back of head on firm surface

And don't forget about the photography tips from Chapter 8. They might come in handy!

# CHAPTER 26.

## HAVE BABY'S HEAD SHAPE EVALUATED

---

While it's not always feasible, ***ideally at the earliest signs of flattening detected by the family or doctor, every baby would receive a head shape evaluation from a clinician skilled in cranial evaluation.***

For many parents, "seeking out a specialist" or "having your child evaluated" are terrifying terms. Deep-breaths, fellow parents. Visiting a helmet provider or a therapist does NOT mean that your baby needs or will receive a helmet or therapy. What it does mean is that a provider with the tools and expertise to take *objective* measurements of your baby's head will tell you the severity of the flattening and help you rule out Torticollis and other contributing factors.

The truth is, most primary care physicians and pediatricians – even really great ones – lack advanced training in and tools for measuring Flat Head Syndrome. "Eyeballing" head shape is difficult and often results in subjective, inaccurate visual assessments of severity and changes over time. Unfortunately, many families are told that their baby's Flat Head Syndrome is mild and their concerns are brushed aside ("let's wait and see"), when in reality the flattening is moderate and getting worse.

*I can nearly guarantee that your child's doctor won't suggest a head shape evaluation from a specialist at the first signs of flattening.* However, many doctors are open to a discussion about the benefits of establishing baseline measurements and getting an objective assessment of severity. ***You are your child's best advocate and have a voice in conversations around how to care for your baby.*** A head shape evaluation may not be available to everyone based on geography and financial limitations, but it is definitely worth considering and looking into.

**Questions to Ask A Specialist:**

- What is the cost of an evaluation?

- Do you accept my insurance? (Also call your insurance provider for specific benefits information.)

- Will I need a physician's referral for an evaluation? (If no, be sure to also ask your insurance provider this question.)

**Ideas for Discussing a Specialist Evaluation With Your Child's Doctor:**

- "I understand that repositioning is an effective way to address head flattening and we are committed to trying that. Measurements of her head shape now and several months from now will help us see if repositioning is helping or not, so I'd like to see a helmet provider to get baseline measurements done."

- "I have concerns and I'd like to be as proactive as possible to make sure my baby's head flattening doesn't get worse. I think having a very clear picture and understanding of her head shape and severity will help us as a family know how to best address this."

# CHAPTER 27.

# IF BABY'S HEAD IS FLAT ACROSS THE BACK

---

If you've noticed your little one's head looking a little flat all the way across the back, now's the time to swing into action with simple strategies to tackle that head flattening.

Your general approach to managing flattening of the whole back of the head through **repositioning** is to DECREASE baby's time with pressure on the back of the head (to stop the progression of Brachycephaly) and INCREASE time with pressure on the sides of the head (to help remold or reshape the head). That's the plan!

I'll give you a heads up, intended to motivate not discourage you. This particular type of flattening can be one of the trickiest to reverse. This is partly because the rounded or bulging parts of the skull that would be most effective to apply pressure to for reshaping the head are the forehead and top of the head. Let's face it, no baby wants to spend any time face-planted on the floor or in a headstand (nor do I recommend those positions)! So we're left with applying pressure to the sides of the head as a way to combat flattening across the back. It can still be effective but extremely diligent repositioning is needed.

Let's use that same Positioning Pyramid concept to develop a plan for emphasizing certain positions while minimizing others.

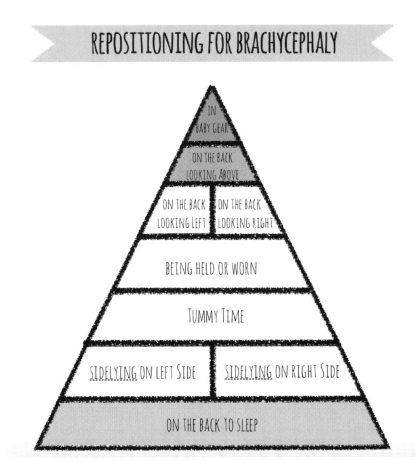

# REPOSITIONING FOR BRACHYCEPHALY

IN BABY GEAR

ON THE BACK LOOKING ABOVE

ON THE BACK LOOKING LEFT | ON THE BACK LOOKING RIGHT

BEING HELD OR WORN

TUMMY TIME

SIDELYING ON LEFT SIDE | SIDELYING ON RIGHT SIDE

ON THE BACK TO SLEEP

Remember that for **Proactive Positioning**, the goal is to combat the effects of the Back to Sleep position. The same general strategies will hold true for managing broad flattening across the back of the head, but you'll want to *be even more diligent with repositioning and even a bit militant in reducing baby's time semi-reclined in baby gear and on the back looking above.* So many parents who've noticed this broad flattening across the back of the head fret and worry each time they lay their baby down in the crib, yet think nothing of lugging their kiddo all over town in an infant car seat carrier. They don't know, but now YOU DO!

Because the day is still 24 hours long (and I do mean LONG when you have an infant at home!), reducing time in Baby

Holding Devices makes more time available for baby to spend in positions that nearly eliminate pressure on the skull and those that place pressure on the sides of the head. Those are the only differences you'll spot in this pyramid if you compare it to the Proactive Positioning Pyramid – the top two sections have shrunk and the middle six sections have increased in size.

## Your Repositioning Toolbox for Brachycephaly

### Sleep

**Diligently follow all Proactive Positioning guidelines for sleep found in Chapter 13.**

**Discuss with your child's doctor the risks and benefits of allowing baby to sleep on her side (alternating sides) or belly (alternating which cheek is down) for supervised naps or for naps on an adult's body (lap, chest, etc.).** For children at lower risk of SIDS, some doctors will support this option for reducing the amount of sleep time spent flat on the back of the head. *Parents must make individual decisions about safe sleep for their babies (and assume all related risks) with full understanding of risks and benefits.*

### Time in Baby Gear

**Reduce time in Baby Holding Devices as much as possible.** In an ideal world, a baby with flattening across the whole back of the head would only be in them for car seat travel in the car.

*In the limited time that baby is in Baby Holding Devices at home,* **strategically position the devices** so that baby is encouraged to turn the head to see what's going on in the room (one side of the device toward a wall). Also, position toys on the sides of the device – alternating to give each side equal time.

*In the limited time that baby is in Baby Holding Devices at home,* use a rolled towel or receiving blanket to prop the head toward one side, alternating to give each side equal time (*exception, do NOT use additional props in a car seat during travel – these may reduce the safety of your baby's seat in the event of a crash).

## Playtime

**Remove all mobiles or nursery decor you may have hanging directly over baby's crib or changing table.** Notice if your baby's usual play spots are under ceiling fans, light fixtures or other decor that might encourage her to look straight up. Strategically choose new play spots that avoid these distractions or position them to the side of baby.

**Reduce the time that baby plays on her back looking directly above.** If you find baby resting on the flat spot even when toys are placed beside her during playtime on the back, create a small wedge to tilt baby's body slightly toward her side. Place a tightly rolled burp cloth, hand towel or receiving blanket under baby's play blanket. Lay baby alongside the "speedbump" you've created with one shoulder and hip propped up slightly and toys placed on the side opposite the roll you've created. Adjust (and entice) as necessary to encourage your sweet babe to turn away from her flat spot. You'll want to alternate which side you prop baby on to promote equal time on her right and left sides.

**Utilize pillows or hats marketed to prevent Flat Head Syndrome for playtimes on the back and for awake time flat in a stroller bassinet or reclined flat stroller seat.** For hats that encourage head turning, be sure to alternate the positioning to promote looking in both directions.

## Wearing and Holding

**Use babywearing as an alternative to Baby Holding Devices** that hold baby in a semi-reclined position – both at home and on the go.

**Hold baby in positions that reduce or eliminate pressure on the back of the head.** Carrying baby in Tummy Time or sidelying, holding in supported sitting and having baby up on your shoulder are great options. Reduce the time you spend holding baby on his back with pressure from your arm, lap or chest directly on the back of his head.

### Daily Care

**Diligently follow Proactive Positioning tips as described in Chapter 22 to promote head turning during diaper changes.**

**Be mindful of feeding positions.** Try to use feeding positions that eliminate pressure directly to the flat area of the head.

### Sitting

**Once baby show signs of readiness for sitting, help baby sit frequently throughout the day.**

**Consider using a baby seat.** If your baby is showing signs of readiness for sitting but isn't yet independently sitting AND doesn't show positional preferences, you might consider using a baby seat that supports him upright for up to an hour per day as an alternative to semi-reclined Baby Holding Devices or lying on his back on the floor. I do not make this same recommendation for babies with flattening on one side of the head or combined Brachycephaly with Plagiocephaly. This is because these babies quite often have some level of asymmetrical preferred positioning that can be exacerbated by baby seats.

# CHAPTER 28.

## IF BABY'S HEAD IS FLATTENING ON ONE SIDE

So your baby's head is getting a little lopsided. I'm so glad you've noticed this issue now because you can get started TODAY making the changes to improve your little one's head shape.

What's your best strategy? To combat flattening on one side of the back of the head through **repositioning**, we'll need to DECREASE baby's time with pressure on that area (to stop the progression of Plagiocephaly) and INCREASE time with pressure on the other areas of the head (to help remold or reshape the head).

Here's how the Positioning Pyramid shifts for babies with asymmetric head flattening. You'll notice that there are now 4 positions at the top of the Pyramid to minimize (shown in gray) and 4 positions in the middle to emphasize (shown in white).

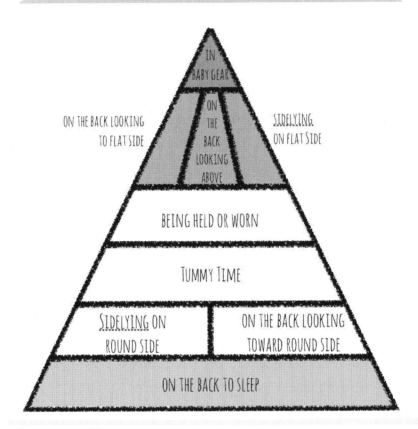

## REPOSITIONING FOR PLAGIOCEPHALY

**IN BABY GEAR**

**ON THE BACK LOOKING TO FLAT SIDE** | **ON THE BACK LOOKING ABOVE** | **SIDELYING ON FLAT SIDE**

**BEING HELD OR WORN**

**TUMMY TIME**

**SIDELYING ON ROUND SIDE** | **ON THE BACK LOOKING TOWARD ROUND SIDE**

**ON THE BACK TO SLEEP**

For the sake of clarity, in this section I'll describe positioning based on your baby's "flat side" and "round side." For example, if your baby has a flat spot on the back right of the head, you'll be reading this section through the lens of "flat side" meaning right and "round side" meaning left. You with me? Let's get to it...

### Your Repositioning Toolbox for Plagiocephaly

### Sleep

**Diligently follow all Proactive Positioning guidelines for sleep from Chapter 13 with several modifications.** Instead of alternating which direction you lay baby in the crib, always position her with a plain wall on her flat side and the door and/or main interest areas of the room on her round side. Mount a crib toy on her round side. Gently position baby's head turned round side toward the mattress each time you put her down to sleep.

**Discuss with your child's doctor the risks/benefits of allowing baby to sleep on her side (round side down) or belly (head turned with cheek on her flat side down) for supervised naps or for naps on an adult's body (lap, chest, etc.).** For children at lower risk of SIDS, some doctors will support this option for reducing the amount of sleep time spent flat on the back of the head. *Parents must make individual decisions about safe sleep for their babies (and assume all related risks) with full understanding of risks and benefits.*

## Time In Baby Gear

**Reduce time in Baby Holding Devices as much as possible.**

*In the limited time that baby is in Baby Holding Devices at home,* **strategically position the devices** so that baby is encouraged to turn the head away from the flat side to see what's going on in the room. Orient devices with a wall on the flat side and the action of the room on the round side. Remove toys from the flat side and, if possible, position toys on baby's round side.

*In the limited time that baby is in Baby Holding Devices at home,* **use a rolled towel or receiving blanket to prop the head turned toward the round side** (*exception, do NOT use additional props in a car seat during travel – these may reduce the safety of your baby's seat in the event of a crash). For travel in the car, use toys, window clings or stickers or an adult in the back seat (when practical) on baby's round side.

**Strategically hang toys in baby's stroller and on Baby Holding Devices** to encourage head turning toward the round side.

**position baby when her stroller is parked.** Take her out of the stroller to hold or wear her. Or take full advantage of a bassinet stroller or flat-reclined stroller seat to emphasize time in sidelying (round side down, flat side up) or Tummy Time.

## Playtime

**Strategically place mobiles or nursery decor near baby's crib or changing table on baby's round side.**

**Strategically choose new play spots that orient ceiling fans, light fixtures and other distracting decor on baby's round side.**

**Hang toys from baby's activity gym on her round side.** For visual exploration, also consider positioning baby beside her activity gym with the whole contraption on her round side.

**During cheek-down Tummy Time, encourage or gently help baby find a resting position with the cheek on the flat side down.** This will apply pressure to that side of the forehead, which is prone to shifting forward and bulging.

**Reduce the time that baby plays on her back looking toward her flat side.** If you find baby resting on the flat spot even when toys are placed beside her during playtime on the back, create a small wedge to tilt baby's body slightly toward her round side. Place a tightly rolled burp cloth, hand towel or receiving blanket under baby's play blanket. Lay baby alongside the "speedbump" you've created with the shoulder and hip on her flat side propped up slightly and toys placed on her round side. Adjust (and entice) as necessary to encourage your sweet babe to turn away from her flat side.

**Utilize pillows or hats marketed to prevent Flat Head Syndrome for playtimes on the back and for awake time flat in a stroller bassinet or reclined flat stroller seat.** For hats that encourage head turning, be sure to follow directions closely in order to encourage turning toward baby's round side.

### Wearing and Holding

**Consistently hold baby in positions that eliminate pressure on the flat side and place pressure on the round side**: in sidelying with the flat side up (round side against your arm) and in Tummy Time with cheek on the same side as flat spot in your hand.

**Wear your baby as an alternative to time in Baby Holding Devices.** Encourage head turning in the same direction as the flat side when baby is worn facing caregiver. For very young babies, you can gently position the head this direction. For older babies, attaching a teether toy to the strap of your carrier, sling or wrap on the same side as baby's round side can encourage this head position.

### Daily Care

**Follow Proactive Positioning tips for diaper changes from Chapter 22 with this modification:** instead of alternating sides of toys or pictures to promote equal head turning, consistently place these objects on baby's round side. Or, place baby on the changing table in the direction that makes YOU (or other super interesting-to-look at caregivers) on baby's round side.

**If bottle feeding, hold baby in whichever of your arms corresponds to her flat side.** For example, for right side flattening, feed with baby held in the crook or elbow of your right arm. This places more pressure on her round side.

### Sitting

**Once baby show signs of readiness for sitting, help baby sit frequently throughout the day and transition to a full**

**upright position in the stroller when awake.**

# CHAPTER 29.

# IF BABY'S HEAD IS FLAT ACROSS THE BACK AND ON ONE SIDE

---

If your baby's head shape seems to be both flat across the back *and* flatter on one side, there's a *Flat Head Syndrome Fix* for you, too. As you can imagine, the tools in your Repositioning Toolbox for this challenge will be a blend of those for each of the two types of flattening your little one is experiencing. Also, the Repositioning Pyramid that will best guide you is the same one from last chapter (labeled 'Repositioning for Plagiocephaly').

By now, you might be beginning to think for yourself of which positions might be best for your baby and even of some **repositioning** strategies you might use. Hoorah! That's the whole goal of this book – to give you the complete understanding of Flat Head Syndrome that you need to find strategies that work for your baby!

As you can probably guess, the emphasis of your diligent repositioning efforts will be on DECREASING pressure on the back of the head, *especially* baby's flat side and INCREASING time spent with pressure on baby's round side. And as usual, your tools are the positions you lay your baby in and the items in your baby's environment that promote independent head turning.

# Your Repositioning Toolbox for Brachycephaly With Plagiocephaly

## Sleep

**Diligently follow all Proactive Positioning guidelines for sleep from Chapter 13 with several modifications.** Instead of alternating which direction you lay baby in the crib, always position her with a plain wall on her flat side and the door and/or main interest areas of the room on her round side. Mount a crib toy on her round side. Gently position baby's head turned round side toward the mattress each time you put her down to sleep.

**Discuss with your child's doctor the risks/benefits of allowing baby to sleep on her side (round side down) or belly (head turned with cheek on her flat side down) for supervised naps or for naps on an adult's body (lap, chest, etc.).** For children at lower risk of SIDS, some doctors will support this option for reducing the amount of sleep time spent flat on the back of the head. *Parents must make individual decisions about safe sleep for their babies (and assume all related risks) with full understanding of risks and benefits.*

## Time in Baby Gear

**Reduce time in Baby Holding Devices as much as possible.** In an ideal world, your baby would only be in them for car seat travel in the car.

*In the limited time that baby is in Baby Holding Devices at home,* **strategically position the devices** so that baby is encouraged to turn the head toward his round side to see what's going on in the room. Orient devices with a wall on the flat side and the action of the room on the round side. Remove toys from the flat side and, if possible, position toys on baby's round side.

*In the limited time that baby is in Baby Holding Devices at home,* use a rolled towel or receiving blanket to prop the head away toward the round side (*exception, do NOT use additional props in a car seat during travel – these may reduce the safety of your baby's seat in the event of a crash). For travel in the car, use toys, window clings or stickers or an adult in the back seat (when practical) on baby's round side.

**Strategically hang toys on baby's round side in a stroller bassinet attachment or flat-reclined stroller seat.**

**Reposition baby when her stroller is parked.** Take her out of the stroller to hold or wear her. Or take full advantage of a bassinet stroller or flat-reclined stroller seat to emphasize time in sidelying (round side down, flat side up) or Tummy Time.

### Playtime

**Strategically choose play spots that orient ceiling fans, light fixtures and other distracting decor on baby's round side.**

**Hang toys from baby's activity gym only on baby's round side.** For visual exploration, also consider positioning baby beside her activity gym with the toys to encourage head turning toward her round side.

**Reduce the time that baby plays on her back looking toward her flat side.** If you find baby resting on the flat spot even when toys are placed beside her during playtime on the back, create a small wedge to tilt baby's body slightly toward her round side. Place a tightly rolled burp cloth, hand towel or receiving blanket under baby's play blanket. Lay baby alongside the "speedbump" you've created with the shoulder and hip on her flat side propped up slightly and toys placed on her round side. Adjust (and entice) as necessary to encourage your sweet babe to turn away from her flat side.

**Utilize pillows or hats marketed to prevent Flat Head**

**Syndrome for playtimes** on the back and for awake time flat in a stroller bassinet or flat-reclined stroller seat. When using hats marketed to promote head turning and reduce flattening, be sure to follow directions in order to encourage turning toward the round side and away from the flat spot.

**During cheek-down Tummy Time, encourage or gently help baby find a resting position with the cheek on her flat side down.** This will apply pressure to that side of the forehead, which is prone to shifting forward and bulging.

### Wearing and Holding

**Consistently hold baby in positions that eliminate pressure on the flat side and place pressure on the round side:** in sidelying with the flat side up (round side against your arm) and in Tummy Time with cheek on same side as flat spot in your hand.

**Wear your baby as an alternative to time in Baby Holding Devices.** Encourage head turning in the same direction as the flat side when baby is worn facing caregiver. For very young babies, you can gently position the head this direction. For older babies, attaching a teether toy to the strap of your carrier, sling or wrap on the same side as baby's round side can encourage this head position.

### Daily Care

**Follow Proactive Positioning tips for diaper changes from Chapter 22 with this modification:** instead of alternating sides of toys or pictures to promote equal head turning, consistently place these objects on baby's round side. Or, place baby on the changing table in the direction that makes YOU (or other super interesting-to-look at caregivers) on baby's round side.

**If bottle feeding, hold baby in whichever of your arms**

**corresponds to her flat side.** For example, for right side flattening, feed with baby held in the crook or elbow of your right arm. This places more pressure on her round side.

### Sitting

**Once baby show signs of readiness for sitting, help baby sit frequently** throughout the day and transition baby to a fully upright stroller position when awake.

CHAPTER 30.

# IF BABY'S HEAD IS NARROW AND LONG

Managing a long, narrow head shape requires a completely different approach than the other three types of head flattening. So while you've dutifully read through all of the positions in the Proactive Positioning Pyramid to learn more about them, I'll now ask that you forget about the strategies that went along with each one. This head shape is a whole new ballgame!

By this point in the book, you may already be thinking, "Bring on the Baby Holding Devices and Back to Sleep positions – those will flatten the back of my baby's head back out in no time!" But wait – there are a few things we need to consider.

The first is that even in the semi-reclined position supported by Baby Holding Devices and on the back for sleep, elongated and narrow heads tend to roll to the side – toward the areas of flattening. This head shape effectively has a fulcrum in the back, and external support is often needed to keep the head centered.

The second consideration is how important movement and position changes are for infant development. Repositioning for the Scaphocephalic head shape becomes a delicate balance of trying to stabilize the head in the middle to INCREASE pressure on the area of roundness or bulging and DECREASING pressure on the flattened sides of the head *while still allowing baby plenty of time to freely move and explore.*

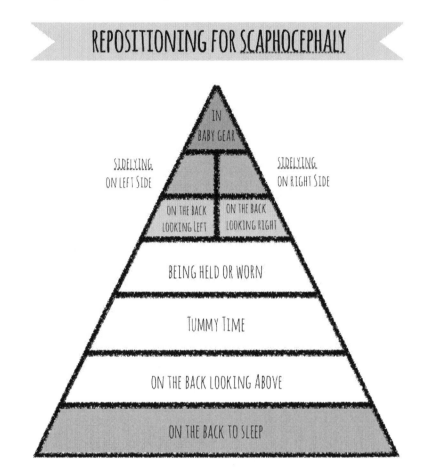

REPOSITIONING FOR SCAPHOCEPHALY

- IN BABY GEAR
- SIDELYING ON LEFT SIDE / SIDELYING ON RIGHT SIDE
- ON THE BACK LOOKING LEFT / ON THE BACK LOOKING RIGHT
- BEING HELD OR WORN
- TUMMY TIME
- ON THE BACK LOOKING ABOVE
- ON THE BACK TO SLEEP

**Your Repositioning Toolbox for Scaphocephaly**

**Sleep**

Add a mobile or other nursery decor directly above your baby's crib or sleeping space.

Keep the wall beside baby's sleeping space blank and free of decor.

Do not use crib toys attached to either side of the crib.

Discuss with your child's doctor the risks/benefits of allowing baby to sleep with external head support (such as rolled receiving blankets secured underneath a fitted crib sheet or a "nest" made from a blanket) for supervised naps or for naps on an adult's body (lap, chest, etc.). For children at lower risk of SIDS, some doctors will support this option for helping increase pressure on the back of the head. *Parents must make individual decisions about safe sleep for their babies (and assume all related risks) with full understanding of risks and benefits.*

### Time in Baby Gear

You still want to limit time in baby gear for your little one's overall development but, with the following repositioning strategies you can stick with an average 2 hour daily maximum.

**Use infant head rest cushions or tightly rolled receiving blankets, burp cloths or hand towels to help support baby's head in the center when in Baby Gear** (exception, do NOT use additional props in a car seat during travel – these may reduce the safety of your baby's seat in the event of a crash).

**Use toy bars on baby gear that position toys directly in front of your baby.** Remove toys from the sides of baby holding devices and strollers.

**If using a bassinet stroller attachment or flat-reclined stroller seat, hang a toy directly above baby if possible.** Use infant head rest cushions or make a "nest"(bunched around the outside of a circle but hollowed out in the middle) from a blanket to support the head in a centered position.

**Hang a soft toy from the head rest or seat back directly in front of baby's car seat** for travel in the car.

### Playtime

**Emphasize playtime on the back with toys directly above baby.** An activity gym, mobiles and an engaging familiar face are all wonderful tools for this.

**Don't avoid sidelying and on the back with head turned positions completely but minimize them** in comparison to time on the back with toys above.

**Place baby's play spot directly under ceiling fans, windows and other pieces of decor** that capture her attention.

**Help baby enjoy playtime while looking directly above her.** If baby's head consistently rolls to the side and stays there during belly-up playtime, create a "nest" out of a blanket to help support baby's head in a centered position.

**Encourage neck strengthening in belly-up play positions by moving a toy or a familiar face very slowly side to side for baby to follow.** Or, use noises, touch and movement of the arm or leg to encourage baby to turn toward what he senses. Strengthening the neck will improve baby's ability to hold the head in the center and overcome the fulcrum effect of her head shape.

### Wearing and Holding

**If baby is old enough to have steady head control, she can be worn facing away from the wearer,** which will place pressure on the back of the head against a caregiver's chest. Just be sure to find a carrier that continues to provide full support of the thigh (avoiding dangling legs).

**Emphasize holding positions that place pressure on the back of baby's head or eliminate pressure on the head completely:** on the back with head against your forearm, upright in a seated position on your arms facing out, belly-up on your thighs looking at you, high on the shoulder with head lifted, etc.

## Daily Care

**Hang a mobile or interesting piece of nursery decor directly above baby's changing table.**

**Leave a blank wall beside baby's changing table.**

**If possible, adjust feeding positions to emphasize pressure on the back of the head.** If bottle-feeding, feeding in the crook of the arm or elbow with nose pointed up can provide this pressure.

## Sitting

**Once baby shows signs of readiness for sitting, help her sit frequently throughout the day** and transition baby to a fully upright stroller position when awake.

# CHAPTER 31.

## DOES MY BABY NEED A HELMET?

---

"Does he really need a helmet?"

"Will a helmet fix it?"

"Will his head round back out on its own?"

"Won't a helmet bother him?"

"Will people stare at her or think there's something really wrong with my baby?"

Stressed out about whether or not to get a helmet for your baby? You are not alone! And odds are, these are just a few of the questions on repeat in your head lately. The decision of whether or not to get a helmet for your baby seems to be particularly agonizing because it taps into some of our biggest fears as parents – a lack of clear answers and guaranteed results, our baby looking different, questioning or judgement from others and possibly making our little one uncomfortable.

Here are some key factors to consider as you try to work through this tricky decision.

### Natural Improvements With Time

After babyhood, head shapes do tend to improve

slightly.[14] There is really no way to know if your child will fit that trend and, if so, how much improvement you might see. But it can be important to consider that your child's head shape may get at least a little bit better after babyhood.

**Severity**

Of course how severely misshapen your baby's head is right now will be your biggest consideration. The most important thing is to receive head shape measurements from a specialist, typically an Orthotist, Craniofacial Doctor, Neurologist or pediatric therapist specializing in head shape issues of infancy. These measurements might be acquired with a high-tech scanner or from hand-measurements using specialized tools. Either way, the experience and skill of the clinician is the biggest factor in accuracy.

These measurements and the expertise of a specialist will help you understand the severity of your child's head flattening. Until you have an evaluation from a specialist, you won't have enough information about your baby's head shape to confidently decide whether or not to pursue a helmet (despite your pediatrician, neighbor and mother-in-law's best proclamations that, "It doesn't look that bad," or "I've seen worse.").

A few things factor into how severity of Flat Head Syndrome is determined, including whether or not there is asymmetry of your baby's facial features. Because asymmetry of the eyes, jaws and ears can have long term health impacts as discussed in Chapter One, it's important to weigh these factors carefully. In fact, *I suggest that the degree of facial asymmetry should be one of the the biggest consideration for parents*.

**Age and Milestones of the Baby**

Typically, parents are faced with the helmeting dilemma when their little one is between 5 and 10 months of age. The younger the baby, the more effective helmet treatment can be.[17] Younger babies have more skull growth ahead of them, and it's that growth that really fuels rapid head shape change. Just to make things a little more confusing (just what you need, right?), **repositioning** is also more effective at younger ages because babies are less active and mobile and still dependent on adults for positioning. In fact, many of the developmental considerations of whether or not to get a helmet are two-sided and a bit confusing. So let's walk through them together.

If your baby is very often rolling out of your attempts to reposition her, very commonly seen around 5 months of age, you can expect that **repositioning** strategies will be less and less effective in the coming weeks and months. However, your baby is likely also more active in her sleep and may even be rolling to sleep on her side or belly (Back to Sleep / Safe to Sleep guidelines advise you to continue to place her on her back for sleep but allow her to sleep in other positions she gets into herself after you put her down). Once your baby is sitting, *if you give her plenty of time to sit upright and stop using Baby Holding Devices other than the car seat for travel*, the progression of Flat Head Syndrome tends to slow down. In light of all of this, take a few days to observe what positions your baby seems to work her way into the most – when awake and asleep.

If your little one is actively working out of **repositioning** strategies and you find her choosing to spend much of her time in positions that continue to put pressure on her flat spot, a helmet is likely the most effective way to change her head shape. If your baby is still responsive to **repositioning** strategies and you feel confident in your ability to stay diligent with them, you might take more time to see how your efforts continue to impact her head shape over time and revisit the helmet decision in a month or two. Especially in light of the next factor...

**The Data You've Collected**

Remember how I said that many, many parents face the helmeting decision with more confidence because they've been monitoring their babies' head shape over time with weekly head checks? I can't stress enough how grateful parents are for the data they've been keeping!

If you've been following *The Flat Head Syndrome Fix*, you very likely have photographs and maybe even measurements that track how your little one's head shape has changed over time and responded to **repositioning**. If you see that your baby's head shape has gotten worse or stayed the same, you can extrapolate that you're not likely to see great improvements going forward and you might be more inclined to pursue a helmet. If you've seen your baby's flat spots rounding out over time, you can be more confident that things may continue to improve even without a helmet. This might motivate you to delay making the helmet decision now and see if the trend continues for another month or two.

**Torticollis**

There's that tricky word again! If your little one has Torticollis or other muscle tightness that hasn't yet resolved when you're presented with the decision of whether or not to use a helmet, this is a *huge* consideration. It puts your baby at a much greater risk of increased flattening over the coming months because those preferred positions are still present.

**"Real Life" Factors**

Does your family life dictate that your baby spends a lot of time riding in her car seat? Does your child attend a daycare that hasn't been on board with your repositioning strategies or requests to limit time in baby gear? Is your little one particularly fussy or does she have a medical condition that limits positioning or mobility? Now that you fully understand Flat Head Syndrome, what contributes to it and what fixes it, you're much better equipped to consider these and other "real life" factors that will likely impact whether your baby's head shape gets better or worse without a helmet.

## Appearance

When it comes to our babies, I'm not one to sweep cosmetic concerns under the rug. Sometimes the difficult decision to get a helmet is largely based on appearance, and there is nothing wrong with that. Parents frequently opt to put braces on their kids' teeth for cosmetic reasons. A non-invasive and pain-free device like a helmet is a similar tool. *Because you are making a healthcare decision on behalf of another person (the most precious person in the world to you), whether or not he'll struggle with self-image because of his head shape when he gets older is a legitimate worry.*

You may choose to consider the gender of your child – many parents of girls worry less about appearance because they anticipate hair covering their daughter's head shape. Another factor to consider is whether your child's head shape might make it hard to fit athletic helmets or glasses (if ear or eye asymmetry is an issue). Because facial asymmetry is often a bigger aesthetic concern to parents than flatness of the back of the head, I suggest again that it should be one of the biggest considerations for parents.

## Cost

Helmets aren't cheap! Without insurance coverage, they typically cost between $2500 and $5000. Many insurances will offer at least partial coverage if certain criteria are met (often based on measurements and a trial of 2 months of **repositioning**).

Another consideration is that babies who experience significant head growth or babies with particularly severe or persistent head flattening are sometimes recommended to get a second helmet to continue treatment. Many parents then face a second agonizing decision of whether to stop treatment and risk regression or continue at a high price.

Finding out the specifics of your insurance coverage or other available funding resources (some families fundraise to cover the cost of a helmet), can help you face your decision with more confidence.

### Commitment

Typically, helmets are to be worn 23 hours a day (one hour off for bathing and daily care) for several months. There are typically many follow-up appointments with your helmet provider for re-measuring and adjusting to accommodate your baby's head growth. Parents' and caregivers' dedication to keeping the helmet on and keeping up with appointments is essential for the best helmet outcomes. If you live 2 hours from the nearest helmet provider or one of your child's caregivers has already said that she won't keep the helmet on, those are really valid things to consider before investing in a helmet.

In general, babies tolerate helmets very well. That said, they tend to get hot more easily when they wear them (your provider can give you tips for keeping your baby cool), some redness or minor rashes are not uncommon and parents are often instructed to remove a helmet if a baby has a fever. So, if you do pursue a helmet, be prepared for your baby to be relatively unphased by it but for you as a parent to face a few bumps or inconveniences along the way.

### Guilt

The reality is that feeling guilty about your baby's head shape is a factor that motivates many parents to pursue a helmet. Remember that your baby didn't come with an instruction manual. Maybe you're faced with the option of helmeting because you didn't know about **repositioning** strategies like those in *The Flat Head Syndrome Fix* early on or you were told to "wait and see." Maybe despite diligent **repositioning**, your baby was one of those with especially severe or particularly persistent head flattening. Perhaps extenuating life or health circumstances made diligent **repositioning** a challenge. I truly believe that nearly every parent tries to do what's best for his or her child using available knowledge. Despite your guilty feelings, isn't that true in your case?

You now have so much knowledge about Flat Head Syndrome – what can make it better and what can make it worse. You have a long list of things to consider before rushing or feeling pushed into a decision about whether or not to get a helmet for your baby. Whether your pediatrician happens to be "anti-helmet" or "pro-helmet" (it can be a divisive topic) and despite the best recommendation of a specialist – the choice is ultimately yours.

Take a few days or weeks to really think through the decision. Process it with your partner or close friends and family. Reach out to people you know who have faced this decision. And, ultimately, make some space and take the time to truly listen to your gut. That's not the clear-cut, cookie cutter answer you're probably craving, but it truly is my best recommendation. It has helped many parents come to a confident decision about whether or not to use a helmet to correct their baby's head shape.

# CONCLUSION

I sit writing the end of this book one month away from my due date with my second child. While the information and strategies I've shared in *The Flat Head Fix* have been part of my professional world for years, they've taken on new personal relevance as I've become a mother.

Just like you, I'm trying to strategize how to put the tools in my "toolbox" into practice as we welcome a new itty bitty squishy baby into our home. And like you, I'm asking myself questions like, "How will I limit time in Baby Holding Devices while keeping baby safe from our dog and a curious toddler sibling?" and "How will I remember to do weekly head shape checks in those chaotic early weeks?"

*The Flat Head Syndrome Fix* isn't prescriptive or one-size-fits-all. It is a set of principles that can provide you with a framework for understanding and impacting your baby's head shape. With a solid understanding of how to use positioning to prevent and manage head flattening, you now have the freedom to get creative and find what works for your baby and your family.

Whether you just had a baby or are expecting one soon, whether your baby's head is nice and round or you've noticed a flat spot forming, **you now have the information and tools you need to impact your little one's head shape**. Some parents will swing into action and put nearly all of the positioning strategies in their newly packed "toolbox" into practice. For others, a few simple changes will bring balance to their babies' "positioning diet" and make a big impact. Ultimately, you have to find what works for your family and for your baby.

Having a new baby can be terrifying and overwhelming. Few of us feel confident that we know what we're doing day in and day out! My biggest wish for you is that you would feel less uncertainty, less worry and more confidence in giving your baby the healthiest start possible. My other wish is that if you found this book helpful, that you would share the resource with other parents. There is a disconnect between what research and clinicians' experience show fights Flat Head Syndrome and the information that parents are receiving. With your help, this book can help bridge that gap.

If you're curious to see *The Flat Head Syndrome Fix* in action and to learn more about your baby's development, visit the blog at CanDoKiddo.com.

# REFERENCES

1. Abbott, A.L., & Bartlett, D.J. (2001). Infant motor development and equipment use in the home. *Child: Care Health and Development, 27,* 295-306.

2. American Academy of Pediatrics, Task Force on Infant Sleep Position and Sudden Infant Death Syndrome (2000). Changing concepts of sudden infant death syndrome: Implications for infant sleeping environment and sleep position. *Pediatrics, 105*(3), 650-656.

3. Bass J.L., & Bull, M. (2002). Oxygen desaturation in term infants in car safety seats. *Pediatrics, 110*(2 pt 1), 401– 402.

4. Bialocerkowski, A. E., Vladusic, S. L., & Ng, C. W. (2008). Prevalence, risk factors, and natural history of positional plagiocephaly: A systematic review. *Developmental Medicine & Child Neurology, 50*(8), 577–86.

5. Biggs, W.S. (2003). Diagnosis and management of positional head deformity. *American Family Physician, 67,* 1953–1956.

6. Biggs, W.S. (2004). The 'Epidemic' of Deformational Plagiocephaly and the American Academy of Pediatrics' Response. *Journal of Prosthetics and Orthotics 16*(4s): 5-8.

7. Boere-Boonekamp, M.M., & Van der Linden-Kuiper, L.T. (2001). Positional Preference: Prevalence in Infants and

Follow-Up After Two Years. *Pediatrics, 107*(2), 339-343.

8. Cabrera-Martos, I., Valenza, M.C., Valenza-Demet, G., Benítez-Feliponi, A., Robles-Vizcaíno, C., & Ruíz-Extremera, A. (2015). Impact of Torticollis Associated With Plagiocephaly on Infants' Motor Development. *Journal of Craniofacial Surgery, 26*(1), 151-156.

9. Callahan, C. W., & Sisler, C. (1997). Use of seating devices in infants too young to sit. *Archives of Pediatric and Adolescent Medicine, 151,* 233–235.

10. Cavalier, A., Picot, M.C., Artiaga, C., Mazurier, E., Amilhau, M.O., Captier, G., Picard, J.C. (2011). Prevention of deformational plagiocephaly in neonates. *Early Human Development, 87,* 537-543.

11. Freed, S.S, & Coulter-O'Berry, C. (2004). Identification and Treatment of Congenital Muscular Torticollis in Infants. *Journal of Prosthetics and Orthotics, 16*(4s), 18-23.

12. Golden, K.A., Beals, S.P., Littlefield, T.R., & Pomatto, J.K. (*1999*) Sternocleidomastoid Imbalance Versus Congenital Muscular Torticollis: Their Relationship to Positional Plagiocephaly. *The Cleft Palate-Craniofacial Journal, 36*(3), 256-261.

13. Hunter, J.G., & Malloy, M.H. (2002). Effect of sleep and play positions on infant development: Reconciling developmental concerns with SIDS prevention. *Newborn and Infant Nursing Reviews, 2*(2), 9-16.

14. Hutchison, B.L, Stewart, A.W., & Mitchell, E.A. (2011). Deformational plagiocephaly: A follow-up of head shape, parental concern and neurodevelopment at ages 3 and 4 years. *Archives of Disease in Childhood, 96,* 85-90.

15. Hutchison, B.L., Thompson, J.M., & Mitchell, E.A. (2003). Determinants of Nonsynostotic Plagiocephaly: A Case-Control Study. *Pediatrics 112*(4), e316.

16. Kane, A.A., Lo, L.J., Vannier, M.W., & Marsh, J.L. (1996). Mandibular dysmorphology in unicoronal synostosis and plagiocephaly without synostosis. *Cleft Palate-Craniofacial Journal 33*(5), 418–23.

17. Kelly, K.M., Littlefield, T.R., Pomatto, J.K., Ripley, C.E., Beals, S.P., & Joganic, E.F. (1999). Importance of early recognition and treatment of deformational plagiocephaly with orthotic cranioplasty. The *Cleft Palate-Craniofacial Journal, 36*(2),127–130.

18. Kordestani, R.K., Patel, S., Bard, D.E., Gurwitch, R. & Panchal, J. (2006). Neurodevelopmental delays in children with deformational plagiocephaly. *Plastic and Reconstructive Surgery 117*(1), 207–18.

19. Laughlin, J., Luerssen, T.G., & Dias, M.S. (2011). Prevention and Management of Positional Skull Deformities in Infants. *Pediatrics, 128*(6), 1236-1241.

20. Littlefield, T.R., Kelly, K.M., & Reiff J.L. (2003). Car seats, infant carriers, and swings: their role in deformational plagiocephaly. *Journal of Prosthetics and Orthotics, 15,* 102–106.

21. Long, T., & Toscano, K. (2002). *Handbook of Pediatric Physical Therapy, second edition.* Philadelphia, PA: Lippincott Williams & Wilkins.

22. Mawji, A., Vollman, A.R., Hatfield, J., McNeil, D.A., & Sauve, R. (2013). The Incidence of Positional Plagiocephaly: A cohort study. *Pediatrics, 132*(2), 298-304.

23. Merchant, J.R., Worwa, C., Porter, S., Coleman, J.M., &

deRegnier, R.A. (2001). Respiratory instability of term and near term healthy newborn infants in car safety seats. *Pediatrics, 108*(3), 647–652.

24. Miller R.I., & Clarren, S.K. (2000). Long-Term Developmental Outcomes in Patients With Deformational Plagiocephaly. *Pediatrics 105*(2), e26.

25. Moon, R.Y. & The American Academy of Pediatrics, Task Force on Infant Sleep Position and Sudden Infant Death Syndrome (2011). SIDS and other sleep-related infant deaths: Expansion of recommendations for a safe infant environment. *Pediatrics, 128*(5), 1341-1367.

26. Panchal, J., Amirsheybani, H., Gurwitch, R., Cook, V., Francel, P., Neas, B., & Levine, N. (2001). Neurodevelopment in children with single-suture craniosynostosis and plagiocephaly without synostosis. *Journal of Plastic & Reconstructive Surgery, 108*(6), 1492–1500.

27. Persing, J., James, H., Swanson, J., Kattwinkel, J. (2003). Prevention and management of positional skull deformities in infants. *Pediatrics, 112*(1), 199-202.

28. Purzycki, A., E., Thompson, L., Argenta, L., & David, L. (2009). Incidence of otitis media in children with deformational plagiocephaly. *Journal of Craniofacial Surgery 20*(5),1407–11.

29. Rogel, P. (2011, June). Torticollis and Plagiocephaly: A Puzzle With Many Pieces. Retrieved from http://www.healio.com/orthotics-prosthetics/diseases-conditions/news/print/o-and-p-news/%7B864f87f6-9c30-456f-a05e-ef03670d7bc8%7D/torticollis-and-plagiocephaly-a-puzzle-with-many-pieces

30. Siatkowski, R.M., Fortney, A.C., Nazir, S.A., Cannon, S.L., Panchal, J., Francel, P., Feuer, W., & Ahmad, W. (2005). Visual

Field Defects in Deformational Posterior Plagiocephaly. *Journal of American Association for Pediatric Ophthalmology and Strabismus, 9*(3), 274-278.

31. St. John, D., Mulliken, J.B., Kaban, L.B., & Padwa, B.L. (2002). Anthropometric analysis of mandibular asymmetry in infants with deformational posterior plagiocephaly. *Journal of Oral and Maxillofacial Surgery, 60*(8), 873-877.

32. Stellwagen, L., Hubbard, E., Chambers, C., & Jones, K.L. (2008). Torticollis, facial asymmetry and plagiocephaly in normal newborns. *Archives of Disease in Childhood, 93*(10): 827-31.

Made in the USA
San Bernardino, CA
28 February 2020